Lecture Notes in Computer Science 10552

Commenced Publication in 1973
Founding and Former Series Editors:
Gerhard Goos, Juris Hartmanis, and Jan van Leeuwen

More information about this series at http://www.springer.com/series/7412

M. Jorge Cardoso · Tal Arbel et al. (Eds.)

Intravascular Imaging and Computer Assisted Stenting, and Large-Scale Annotation of Biomedical Data and Expert Label Synthesis

6th Joint International Workshops, CVII-STENT 2017
and Second International Workshop, LABELS 2017
Held in Conjunction with MICCAI 2017
Québec City, QC, Canada, September 10–14, 2017
Proceedings

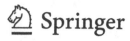 Springer

Editors
M. Jorge Cardoso
University College London
London
UK

Tal Arbel
McGill University
Montreal, QC
Canada

Workshop Editors *see next page*

ISSN 0302-9743   ISSN 1611-3349   (electronic)
Lecture Notes in Computer Science
ISBN 978-3-319-67533-6   ISBN 978-3-319-67534-3   (eBook)
DOI 10.1007/978-3-319-67534-3

Library of Congress Control Number: 2017953390

LNCS Sublibrary: SL6 – Image Processing, Computer Vision, Pattern Recognition, and Graphics

Printed on acid-free paper

This Springer imprint is published by Springer Nature
The registered company is Springer International Publishing AG
The registered company address is: Gewerbestrasse 11, 6330 Cham, Switzerland

Workshop Editors

6th Joint International Workshops on Computing and Visualization for Intravascular Imaging and Computer Assisted Stenting, CVII-STENT 2017

Su-Lin Lee
Imperial College London
London
UK

Stefanie Demirci
Technical University Munich
Munich
Germany

Simone Balocco
University of Barcelona
Barcelona
Spain

Luc Duong
École de Technologie Supérieure
Montreal, QC
Canada

Guillaume Zahnd
Nara Institute of Science and Technology
Nara
Japan

Shadi Albarqouni
Technical University Munich
Munich
Germany

Second International Workshop on Large-Scale Annotation of Biomedical Data and Expert Label Synthesis, LABELS 2017

Veronika Cheplygina 🆔
Eindhoven University of Technology
Eindhoven
The Netherlands

Eric Granger
École de Technologie Supérieure
Montreal, QC
Canada

Diana Mateus
Technical University of Munich
Garching
Germany

Marc-André Carbonneau
École de Technologie Supérieure
Montreal, QC
Canada

Lena Maier-Hein
DKFZ
Heidelberg
Germany

Gustavo Carneiro 🆔
University of Adelaide
Adelaide, SA
Australia

Preface CVII-STENT 2017

MICCAI 2017 is again hosting the Joint MICCAI-Workshops on Computing and Visualization for Intravascular Imaging and Computer Assisted Stenting (MICCAI CVII-STENT), focusing on the technological and scientific research surrounding endovascular procedures. This series of workshops has become an important annual platform for the interchange of knowledge and ideas for medical experts and technological researchers in the field.

This year, we have much to celebrate with the launch earlier this year of the CVII-STENT book, published by Elsevier. Many of the authors have been involved with the workshop since its infancy and continue to be part of this research community.

We look forward to this year's invited talks and presentations on the state of the art in imaging, treatment, and computer-assisted interventions in the field of endovascular interventions. We also extend our thanks to the reviewers, who have helped ensure the high quality of the papers presented at CVII-STENT.

September 2017

Su-Lin Lee
Simone Balocco
Guillaume Zahnd
Stefanie Demirci
Luc Duong
Shadi Albarqouni

Organization

Organizing Committee

Su-Lin Lee	Imperial College London, UK
Simone Balocco	University of Barcelona, Spain
Guillaume Zahnd	Nara Institute of Science and Technology, Japan
Stefanie Demirci	Technical University of Munich, Germany
Luc Duong	École de technologie supérieure, Canada
Shadi Albarqouni	Technical University of Munich, Germany

Steering Committee

Petia Radeva	University of Barcelona, Spain
Markus Kowarschik	Siemens Healthcare, Germany
Amin Katouzian	IBM Almaden Research Center, USA
Gabor Janiga	Otto-von-Guericke Universität Magdeburg, Germany
Ernst Schwartz	Medical University Vienna, Austria
Marcus Pfister	Siemens Healthcare, Germany
Simon Lessard	Centre hospitalier de l'Université de Montréal (CHUM), Canada
Jouke Dijkstra	Leiden University Medical Center, Netherlands

Industrial Committee

Ying Zhu	Siemens Corporate Research, USA
Regis Vaillant	General Electric, France
Amin Katouzian	IBM Almaden Research Center, USA
Heinz Kölble	Endoscout GmbH, Germany
Torsten Scheuermann	Admedes Schuessler GmbH, Germany
Frederik Bender	piur imaging GmbH, Germany

Medical Committee

Frode Manstad-Hulaas	St. Olavs Hospital, Norway
Hans-Henning Eckstein	Klinikum rechts der Isar, Germany
Reza Ghotbi	Kreisklinik München-Pasing, Germany
Christian Reeps	Klinikum rechts der Isar, Germany
Mojtaba Sadeghi	Klinikum Landkreis Erding, Germany

Publicity Chair

Stefano Moriconi   University College London, UK

Program Committee

Atefeh Abdolmanafi	CHU Sainte-Justine Research Center, Canada
Christoph Baur	Technische Universität München, Germany
Katharina Breininger	Friedrich-Alexander-Universität Erlangen-Nürnberg, Germany
Anees Kazi	Technische Universität München, Germany
Benjamín Gutiérrez-Becker	Technische Universität München, Germany
Maximilian Baust	Technische Universität München, Germany
Giovanni J. Ughi	Harvard Medical School, USA
Leonardo Flórez-Valencia	Pontificia Universidad Javeriana, Colombia
Salvatore Scaramuzzino	Magna Grecia University, Italy
Angelos Karlas	Technische Universität München, Germany
Ivan Macia	Vicomtech-IK4, Spain
Cristina Oyarzun Laura	Fraunhofer-Institut, Germany
Karen López-Linares Román	Vicomtech-IK4, Spain
Menglong Ye	Hamlyn Centre for Robotic Surgery, London, UK
Pierre Ambrosini	Biomedical Imaging Group Rotterdam, Erasmus MC, Netherlands

Preface LABELS 2017

The second international workshop on Large-scale Annotation of Biomedical data and Expert Label Synthesis (LABELS) was held in Quebec City on September 14th, 2017, in conjunction with the 20th International Conference on Medical Image Computing and Computer Assisted Intervention (MICCAI).

Supervised learning techniques have been of increasing interest to the MICCAI community. However, the effectiveness of such approaches often depends on their access to sufficiently large quantities of labeled data. Despite the increasing amount of clinical data, the availability of ready-to-use annotations is still limited. To address these issues, LABELS gathers contributions and approaches focused on either adapting supervised learning methods to learn from external types of labels (e.g., multiple instance learning, transfer learning) and/or acquiring more, or more informative, annotations, and thus reducing annotation costs (e.g., active learning, crowdsourcing).

Following the success of LABELS 2016, a decision was made to organize the second workshop in 2017. The workshop included three invited talks by Danna Gurari (University of Texas at Austin), Emanuele Trucco (University of Dundee), and Tanveer Syeda-Mahmood (IBM), as well as several contributed papers and abstracts. After peer review, a total of 11 papers and 4 abstracts were selected. The papers appear in this volume, and the abstracts are available for viewing on our website, http://www. labels2017.org. The variety of approaches for dealing with few labels, from transfer learning to crowdsourcing, are well-represented within the workshop. Unlike many workshops, the contributions also feature "insightfully unsuccessful" results, which illustrate the difficulty of collecting annotations in the real world.

We would like to thank all the speakers and authors for joining our workshop, the Program Committee for their excellent work with the peer reviews, our sponsor - understand. AI - for their support, and our advisory committee and the workshop chairs for their help with the organization of the second LABELS workshop.

September 2017

Veronika Cheplygina
Diana Mateus
Lena Maier-Hein
Eric Granger
Marc-André Carbonneau
Gustavo Carneiro

Organization

Organizing Committee

Veronika Cheplygina	Eindhoven University of Technology (TU/e), The Netherlands
Diana Mateus	Technische Universität München (TUM), Germany
Lena Maier-Hein	German Cancer Research Center (DKFZ), Germany
Eric Granger	École de technologie supérieure (ETS), Canada
Marc-André Carbonneau	École de technologie supérieure (ETS), Canada
Gustavo Carneiro	University of Adelaide, Australia

Program Committee

Adrian Barbu	Florida State University, USA
Danna Gurari	University of Texas at Austin, USA
Dinggang Shen	UNC Chapel Hill, USA
Filipe Condessa	Instituto Superior Tecnico, Portugal
Jaime Cardoso	Universidade do Porto, Portugal
Joao Papa	Sao Paulo State University, Brazil
Ksenia Konyushova	EPFL, Switzerland
Le Lu	NIH, USA
Loic Peter	University College London, UK
Marco Pedersoli	École de technologie supérieure, Canada
Michael Goetz	German Cancer Research Center (DKFZ), Germany
Neeraj Dhungel	The University of Adelaide, Australia
Raphael Sznitman	University of Bern, Switzerland
Roger Tam	The University of British Columbia, Canada
Shadi Albarqouni	Technische Universität München, Germany
Silas Ørting	University of Copenhagen, Denmark
Weidong Cai	University of Sydney, Australia

Advisory Board

Marco Loog	Delft University of Technology (TU Delft), The Netherlands

Logo Design

Carolin Feldmann	German Cancer Research Center (DKFZ)

Contents

6th Joint International Workshops on Computing and Visualization for Intravascular Imaging and Computer Assisted Stenting, CVII-STENT 2017

Robust Detection of Circles in the Vessel Contours and Application to Local Probability Density Estimation

Luis Alvarez[1]([⊠]), Esther González[1], Julio Esclarín[1], Luis Gomez[2],
Miguel Alemán-Flores[1], Agustín Trujillo[1], Carmelo Cuenca[1], Luis Mazorra[1],
Pablo G. Tahoces[3], and José M. Carreira[4]

[1] CTIM, Departamento de Informática y Sistemas, Universidad de Las Palmas de Gran Canaria, Las Palmas, Spain
{lalvarez,esther.gonzalez,julio.esclarin,miguel.aleman,
agustin.trujillo,carmelo.cuenca,lmazorra,luis.gomez}@ulpgc.es
[2] CTIM, Dpto. de Ingeniería Electrónica y Automática, Universidad de Las Palmas de Gran Canaria, Las Palmas, Spain
[3] CITIUS, Universidad de Santiago de Compostela, A Coruña, Spain
{pablo.tahoces,josemartin.carreira}@usc.es
[4] Complejo Hospitalario Universitario de Santiago (CHUS), A Coruña, Spain

Abstract. In this work we propose a technique to automatically estimate circular cross-sections of the vessels in CT scans. First, a circular contour is extracted for each slice of the CT by using the Hough transform. Afterward, the locations of the circles are optimized by means of a parametric snake model, and those circles which best fit the contours of the vessels are selected by applying a robust quality criterion. Finally, this collection of circles is used to estimate the local probability density functions of the image intensity inside and outside the vessels. We present a large variety of experiments on CT scans which show the reliability of the proposed method.

Keywords: Vessels · Circle Hough transform · Seed point · Histogram analysis · CT images

1 Introduction

Most of the techniques for the segmentation of vessels require seed points inside the vessels and an analysis of the intensity histogram to separate the vessels from the surrounding tissues. For instance, in [1], the authors use an initial circle inside the aortic lumen and two intensity thresholds for CT images in order to track the geometry of the aortic lumen by using an elliptical model of its cross-sections. In [4], the authors propose a region growing-based strategy for vessel segmentation which starts by manually placing one or more seed points in the vessel(s) of interest. From these seed points, more neighboring voxels are included in the segmentation using some image intensity thresholds. In [7], a

© Springer International Publishing AG 2017
M.J. Cardoso et al. (Eds.): CVII-STENT/LABELS 2017, LNCS 10552, pp. 3–11, 2017.
DOI: 10.1007/978-3-319-67534-3_1

review of 3D techniques for the segmentation of the vessel lumen is presented. In particular, some of the techniques which are studied use probability distribution models of the aorta and the surrounding tissues.

The usual way to automatically compute a seed point inside the vessels consists in using the Hough transform to search for circular vessel contours. In [2], the authors propose the Hough transform to automatically locate a circle in the descending aorta in MR images. In [8], the authors propose to use the most caudal image slice to locate the position of the aorta using the Hough transform. In [9], the authors propose to use the Hough transform to detect the ascending aorta using the prior knowledge about the expected range for the diameter of the ascending aorta (from 22 mm to 34 mm).

In this paper we propose to combine the Hough transform with the following parametric snake model proposed in [6] to estimate accurately circle locations:

$$E(R, \bar{c}) = \frac{1}{2\pi} \int_0^{2\pi} \nabla I_\sigma(C(\theta)) \cdot \bar{n}(\theta) d\theta \tag{1}$$

$$+ \alpha_- \left(\frac{\iint_{A_-} (I_\sigma(C(\theta)) - I_-)^2 r dr d\theta}{|A_-|} \right)^{\frac{1}{2}} + \alpha_+ \left(\frac{\iint_{A_+} (I_\sigma(C(\theta)) - I_+)^2 r dr d\theta}{|A_+|} \right)^{\frac{1}{2}}$$

where $C(\theta) = (c_x + R \cdot cos(\theta), c_y + R \cdot sin(\theta))$, I_σ is the original image convolved with a Gaussian kernel, $\alpha_-, \alpha_+ \geq 0$, A_-, A_+ are annulus in both sides of the circle contour, and I_-, I_+ are the average of I_σ in A_-, A_+. The local minima of this energy correspond to circles which fit high image contrast areas. We point out that, using the Hough transform, the locations of the circle centers and their radii are usually given in integer (or low) precision. Using the circles provided by the Hough transform as initialization, the application of the parametric snake model improves the accuracy of the circle locations and provides a measure of the quality of the circles. The lower the value of $E(R, \bar{c})$, the higher the quality of the circle. In fact, in this paper we combine several circle quality estimators to select the "best" circle along the image slices in a robust way. By measuring the similarity with the "best" circle, we select a collection of circles which correspond to vessel contours. This collection of circles is used to estimate, in a local way, the probability density functions of the intensity inside and outside the vessels by using a kernel density estimation. We point out that these probability distributions are very useful pieces of information for the automatic segmentation of the vessels.

The main contributions of this paper are:

- A new method for the automatic and robust computation of a collection of circular cross-sections of the vessels based on the combination of the Hough transform, a snake parametric model and a new quality criterion for the circle selection. The centers of such circles can be used as seed points for the automatic segmentation of vessels.
- A new technique for the kernel density estimation of the local probability density functions inside and outside the vessels based on the sampling of the image intensity values inside the collection of circles and in a neighborhood

of those circles. We point out that, as the collection of circles is distributed along the slices of the 3D image, by considering a neighborhood around each circle, we obtain a reliable sample of the intensities in a neighborhood of the whole vessel.

The rest of the paper is organized as follows: In Sect. 2, we present the proposed method to compute a collection of circles on the vessel contours. In Sect. 3, we study how to estimate the probability density distributions of the image intensity values inside and outside the vessels. In Sect. 4, we present some experiments and, in Sect. 5, we present the main conclusions.

2   Detection of Circles in the Vessel Contours

Let I be a $3D$ image consisting of N slices. That is, $I = \{I^z\}_{z=1,..,N}$. For each slice I^z, using the circle Hough transform, we compute the most voted circle, C^z, with center (c_x^z, c_y^z) and radius R^z for a range of circle radii in the interval $[R_{min}, R_{max}]$ (in the experiments presented in this paper we use $R_{min} = 5\,\text{mm}$, $R_{max} = 15\,\text{mm}$). The locations of such circles are then optimized to fit the vessel contour by minimizing the energy criterion proposed in [6] (equation (6)) using a parametric snake model. From the collection of circles $\{C^z\}$, we select, in a robust way, the "best" one by combining several quality criteria. The main goal is that the contour of the selected circle belongs to the vessel contour with a high probability. The quality criteria we use are:

1. The voting score V^z, provided by the Hough transform. The higher the value of V^z, the better.
2. The circle energy E^z, provided by the method proposed in [6], which measures how well the circle fits an image contour. The lower the value of E^z, the better.
3. The standard deviation σ^z of the image intensity values I^z inside the circle. We assume that the variation of the image intensity inside the vessel is low, so that the lower the value of σ^z, the better.
4. In general, the location of the circles C^z across the sequence is expected to be stable in the slices of the CT scan where the vessel contours have a circular shape. Therefore, we use the distance D^z between the circle centers (c_x^z, c_y^z) and (c_x^{z+1}, c_y^{z+1}) as quality measure. Since this estimation is very local, we convolve $\{D^z\}$ with a Gaussian kernel to obtain a more reliable estimation. The lower the value of D^z, the better.

Next, we combine the above quality measures in the following way to obtain a robust and reliable circle quality criterion Q^z:

$$Q^z = \frac{V^z}{median\{V^z\}} - \frac{E^z}{median\{E^z\}} - \frac{\sigma^z}{median\{\sigma^z\}} - \frac{D^z}{median\{D^z\}}. \qquad (2)$$

The higher the value of Q^z, the better the circle. Then we select the "best" reference circle $C^{z_{opt}}$ as the one which maximizes Q^z. We observe that we can include different weights as parameters in the combination of the quality criteria in the definition of Q^z. However, to simplify the exposition, in this paper we use the fixed combination given by the above equation.

Once the reference circle $C^{z_{opt}}$ has been obtained, we use it to select, by similarity, a collection of circles $\{C^{z_i}\} \subset \{C^z\}$ which belong to the vessel contours. We assume that C^{z_i} lies entirely inside the vessel if Q^{z_i} is big enough and the mean and standard deviation of the image intensity values inside C^{z_i}, μ^{z_i} and σ^{z_i} respectively, are similar to those for $C^{z_{opt}}$. That is,

$$\{C^{z_i}\} = \{C^z : Q_z > p_Q \text{ and } \frac{|\mu^z - \mu^{z_{opt}}|}{\mu^{z_{opt}}} < p_\mu \text{ and } \frac{|\sigma^z - \sigma^{z_{opt}}|}{median\{\sigma_z\}} < p_\sigma\}, \quad (3)$$

where $p_Q, p_\mu, p_\sigma > 0$ are parameters of the algorithm. We point out that, with the proposed approach, we avoid the detection of circles on non-vascular structures, as shown in the experimental results. Indeed, there exist other organs, like the trachea or the backbone, where the CT cross-sections may have a circular shape. However, with our approach, the circles in the trachea are not selected because they correspond to dark circles surrounded by a brighter background (and the proposed method looks for the opposite, that is, bright circles in a darker background). In the backbone, the standard deviation of the image intensity inside the circle is much higher than in the vessels, so that our quality criterion penalizes such circles with respect to the circles in the vessels.

3   Application to the Local Analysis of the Histogram Around the Vessels

Let $\{C^{z_i}\}$ be the collection of circles in the vessel contours estimated using the proposed method. Given $\lambda > 0$, we define $C_\lambda^{z_i}$ as the circle with the same center as C^{z_i} and area equal to $\lambda \cdot AREA(C^{z_i})$. Based on the collection of circles $\{C_\lambda^{z_i}\}$, we define the sample S_λ, of the image intensity values as

$$S_\lambda = \{I^{z_i}(x) : x \in C_\lambda^{z_i}\}. \quad (4)$$

We use a kernel density estimation (KDE) to approximate the probability density function of the sample S_λ. That is, the kernel density estimator is

$$\hat{f}_h^\lambda(s) = \frac{1}{|S_\lambda|h} \sum_{s_k \in S_\lambda} K\left(\frac{s - s_k}{h}\right), \quad (5)$$

where $K(\cdot)$ is the kernel (in this paper we use the normal distribution $N(0,1)$ as $K(\cdot)$) and h is the bandwidth (in the experiments we fix the value of h to 5). We point out that $\hat{f}_h^1(s)$ is an approximation of the probability density inside the vessels and $\hat{f}_h^2(s)$ is an approximation of the probability density in a local neighborhood of the vessels. Next, from $\hat{f}_h^1(s)$ and $\hat{f}_h^2(s)$, we estimate the probability density of the image intensity values in S_2 outside the vessels, $\hat{g}_h^{1,2}(s)$. First we observe that

$$\hat{f}_h^2(s) = a\hat{f}_h^1(s) + (1-a)\hat{g}_h^{1,2}(s), \quad (6)$$

where $a > 0$, is the proportion of points in S_2 which are inside the vessels. To estimate a, we assume that, locally, there are no points outside the vessels with an intensity value close to the median of the intensity values inside the vessels. That is, we assume that $\hat{g}_h^{1,2}(s) \approx 0$ for $s \in [p_1, p_2]$, where p_1, p_2 are percentile values of $\hat{f}_h^1(s)$ around its median (in the experiments shown in this paper, we use p_1 as the 40th percentile value and p_2 as the 60th percentile value). Then, we estimate a as

$$a = median \left\{ \frac{\hat{f}_h^2(s)}{\hat{f}_h^1(s)} \right\}_{s \in [p_1, p_2]}. \tag{7}$$

Once a is estimated, we approximate $\hat{g}_h^{1,2}(s)$ as

$$\hat{g}_h^{1,2}(s) = \frac{1}{M} \max \left\{ \frac{\hat{f}_h^2(s) - a\hat{f}_h^1(s)}{1 - a}, 0 \right\}, \tag{8}$$

where $M > 0$ is fitted in such a way that $\hat{g}_h^{1,2}(s)$ integrates to one.

4 Experimental Results

First, we study the ability of criterion (2) to obtain robust and reliable circles in the contours of the vessels. To obtain the initial circle in each slice, we use a gradient-based Hough transform which takes into account that, in a CT scan, the intensity values are usually brighter inside the vessels than in the surrounding tissues. For comparison purposes, we also use a standard implementation of the Hough transform. In our dataset, we use 10 high-quality contrast-enhanced MDCT scans provided by the University Hospital Complex of Santiago de Compostela (CHUS) and 332 contrast-enhanced scans from the database LIDC-IDRI (see [3,5]). This database has been designed for lung cancer screening and the images are, in general, of poor quality for our purpose.

In Table 1, we show the region where the reference circle is located when we use the standard Hough circle transform maximizing the voting score, and when we apply the proposed method maximizing the circle quality score Q^z.

Table 1. Location of the reference circle obtained by maximizing the voting score using the standard Hough circle transform, and by using the proposed method maximizing the circle quality score Q^z for the image databases we use.

	aorta	innominate trunk	backbone	trachea	other
Standard Hough (CHUS database)	9	0	1	0	0
Proposed method (CHUS database)	10	0	0	0	0
Standard Hough (LIDC database)	238	1	44	32	17
Proposed method (LIDC database)	324	8	0	0	0

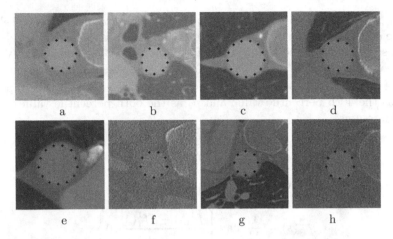

Fig. 1. Circle obtained by maximizing Q^z along the image slices for 8 images of the LIDC-IDRI database.

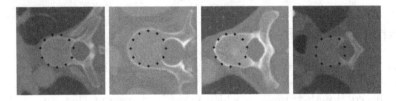

Fig. 2. Examples of images of the LIDC-IDRI database where the circle which maximizes the standard Hough transform is located in the backbone.

We point out that, in the backbone and in the trachea, the image contours may have a circular shape and the standard Hough transform could therefore provide the reference circle in these areas. In a CT scan, the image intensity inside the trachea is darker than outside it, so that the proposed method never selects the trachea contour as circle because we assume that the intensity is brighter inside the circle than outside it in the gradient-based Hough implementation. On the other hand, in the quality criterion Q^z, we consider the standard deviation of the image intensity and the stability of the position of the circle across the sequence. In general, these estimators are lower inside the vessel than in the backbone, which reduces the probability of attaining the minimum of Q^z in the backbone. In Fig. 1, we show the circle obtained by maximizing Q^z along the image slices for 8 CT scans of LIDC-IDRI database. In Fig. 2, we show 4 images of the LIDC-IDRI database where the circle which maximizes the standard Hough transform is located in the backbone. In Fig. 3, we show 4 images of the LIDC-IDRI database where the circle which maximizes the standard Hough transform is located in the trachea. Another limitation of the standard Hough transform is that, in some cases, the circle which maximizes the voting score cannot properly fit the vessel contours. This is illustrated in Fig. 4. This lack of accuracy is solved

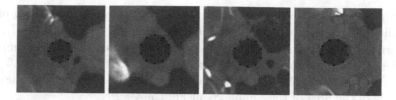

Fig. 3. Examples of images of the LIDC-IDRI database where the circle which maximizes the standard Hough transform is located in the trachea.

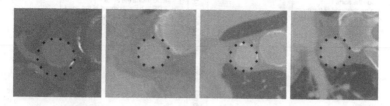

Fig. 4. Examples of images of the LIDC-IDRI database where the circle which maximizes the standard Hough transform does not properly fit the vessel contours.

in the proposed method in 2 ways. On the one hand, we consider the standard deviation of the image intensity inside the circle and, on the other hand, we improve the circle location using the parametric snake model introduced in [6]. In Fig. 5, for one tomography of CHUS database, we show 8 out of 234 circles selected by similarity with the reference one using criterion (3). All 234 circles are inside the vessels, most of them in the aorta. The first selected circle is in the innominate trunk and the last one is in the iliac artery. We point out that we consider that our method works properly if all selected circles are inside the vessels.

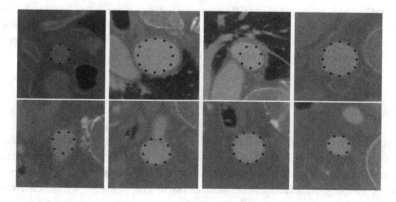

Fig. 5. Examples of some of the 234 circles selected by similarity with the reference one using criterion (3) for one image of the CHUS database.

In Fig. 6, we show, for 4 images of the CHUS database, the KDE of the probability distribution of the image intensity inside the vessels ($\hat{f}_h^1(s)$), in a neighborhood of the vessels ($\hat{f}_h^2(s)$), and outside the vessels ($\hat{g}_h^{1,2}$), computed using the proposed approach. We observe that the value of a is close to 0.5. This is due to the fact that the size of the sample S_2 in the vessel neighborhood is the double of the area of the sample S_1 inside the vessels.

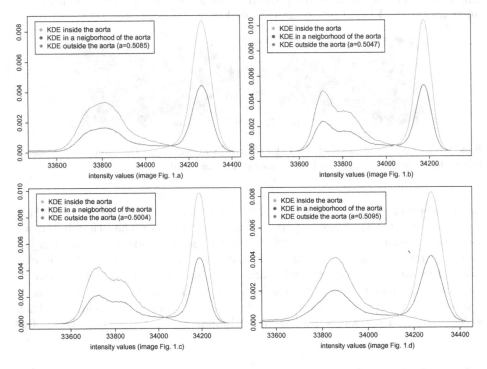

Fig. 6. KDE of the probability distribution of the image intensity inside the vessels, $\hat{f}_h^1(s)$, in a neighborhood of the vessels, $\hat{f}_h^2(s)$, and outside the vessels, $\hat{g}_h^{1,2}(s)$, computed using the proposed approach for 4 images of the CHUS database. For each case, we also show the estimated proportion of vessel points, a, using (7).

5   Conclusions

In this paper we propose a new method for the automatic and robust computation of a collection of circles in the vessel contours and a quality criterion for the circle selection. From this information, we compute the KDE of the local probability density function inside and outside the vessels, which can be very useful in vessel segmentation techniques. Moreover, the centers of the selected circles can be used as seed points inside the vessels. As shown in the experimental results, the Hough transform voting score alone is not a reliable criterion for circle selection. The circle quality criterion proposed in this paper provides a much more robust estimation and the results in a large variety of CT scans are very promising. The shapes of the KDE estimations, shown in Fig. 6, suggest that the usual normal distribution model to approximate the probability distribution inside the vessels is not very accurate. This is likely due to the fact that the image intensity values are lowered near the boundary of the vessels because of the influence of the surrounding tissues.

Acknowledgement. This research has partially been supported by the MINECO projects references TIN2016-76373-P (AEI/FEDER, UE) and MTM2016-75339-P (AEI/FEDER, UE) (Ministerio de Economía y Competitividad, Spain). The authors acknowledge the National Cancer Institute and the Foundation for the National Institutes of Health, and their critical role in the creation of the free publicly available LIDC/IDRI Database used in this study.

References

1. Alvarez, L., Trujillo, A., Cuenca, C., González, E., Esclarín, J., Gomez, L., Mazorra, L., Alemán-Flores, M.G., Tahoces, P., Carreira, J.M.: Tracking the aortic lumen geometry by optimizing the 3D orientation of its cross-sections. In: MICCAI 2017 (2017, to appear)
2. Adame, I.M., van der Geest, R.J., Bluemke, D.A., Lima, J.A., Reiber, J.H., Lelieveldt, B.P.: Automatic vessel wall contour detection and quantification of wall thickness in in-vivo MR images of the human aorta. J. Magn. Reson. Imaging **24**(3), 595–602 (2006)
3. Armato, S.G., et al.: The lung image database consortium (LIDC) and image database resource initiative (IDRI): a completed reference database of lung nodules on CT scans. Med. Phys. **38**(2), 915–931 (2011)
4. Boskamp, T., Rinck, D., Link, F., Kmmerlen, B., Stamm, G., Mildenberger, P.: New vessel analysis tool for morphometric quantification and visualization of vessels in CT and MR imaging data sets. RadioGraphics **24**(1), 287–297 (2004)
5. Clark, K., Vendt, B., Smith, K., Freymann, J., Kirby, J., Koppel, P., Moore, S., Phillips, S., Maffitt, D., Pringle, M., Tarbox, L., Prior, F.: The cancer imaging archive (TCIA): maintaining and operating a public information repository. J. Digit. Imaging **26**(6), 1045–1057 (2013)
6. Cuenca, C., González, E., Trujillo, A., Esclarín, J., Mazorra, L., Alvarez, L., Martínez-Mera, J.A., Tahoces, P.G., Carreira, J.M.: Fast and accurate circle tracking using active contour models. J. Real-Time Image Process. 1–10 (2015)
7. Lesage, D., Angelini, E.D., Bloch, I., Funka-Lea, G.: A review of 3D vessel lumen segmentation techniques: models, features and extraction schemes. Med. Image Anal. **13**(6), 819–845 (2009)
8. Martínez-Mera, J.A., Tahoces, P.G., Carreira, J.M., Suárez-Cuenca, J.J., Souto, M.: A hybrid method based on level set and 3D region growing for segmentation of the thoracic aorta. Comput. Aided Surg. **18**(5–6), 109–117 (2013)
9. Wang, S., Fu, L., Yue, Y., Kang, Y., Liu, J.: Fast and automatic segmentation of ascending aorta in MSCT volume data. In: 2009 2nd International Congress on Image and Signal Processing, pp. 1–5, October 2009

Intra-coronary Stent Localization in Intravascular Ultrasound Sequences, A Preliminary Study

Simone Balocco[1,2](✉), Francesco Ciompi[3,4], Juan Rigla[5], Xavier Carrillo[6], Josepa Mauri[6], and Petia Radeva[1,2]

[1] Department Matematics and Informatics, University of Barcelona,
Gran Via 585, 08007 Barcelona, Spain
balocco.simone@gmail.com
[2] Computer Vision Center, 08193 Bellaterra, Spain
[3] Computational Pathology Group, Department of Pathology,
Radboud University Medical Center, Nijmegen, Netherlands
[4] Diagnostic Image Analysis Group, Department of Radiology
and Nuclear Medicine, Radboud University Medical Center, Nijmegen, Netherlands
[5] InspireMD, Boston, MA, USA
[6] University Hospital Germans Trias I Pujol, 08916 Badalona, Spain

Abstract. An intraluminal coronary stent is a metal scaffold deployed in a stenotic artery during Percutaneous Coronary Intervention (PCI). Intravascular Ultrasound (IVUS) is a catheter-based imaging technique generally used for assessing the correct placement of the stent. All the approaches proposed so far for the stent analysis only focused on the struts detection, while this paper proposes a novel approach to detect the boundaries and the position of the stent along the pullback. The pipeline of the method requires the identification of the stable frames of the sequence and the reliable detection of stent struts. Using this data, a measure of likelihood for a frame to contain a stent is computed. Then, a robust binary representation of the presence of the stent in the pullback is obtained applying an iterative and multi-scale approximation of the signal to symbols using the SAX algorithm. Results obtained comparing the automatic results versus the manual annotation of two observers on 80 IVUS in-vivo sequences shows that the method approaches the inter-observer variability scores.

1 Introduction

An intraluminal coronary stent is a metal mesh tube deployed in a stenotic artery during Percutaneous Coronary Intervention (PCI). Ideally, the stent should be implanted and optimally expanded along the vessel axis, considering vessel anatomical structures such as bifurcations and stenoses.

Intravascular Ultrasound (IVUS) is a catheter-based imaging technique generally used for assessing the correct expansion, aposition and precise placement

---

S. Balocco and F. Ciompi equally contributed to the paper.

© Springer International Publishing AG 2017
M.J. Cardoso et al. (Eds.): CVII-STENT/LABELS 2017, LNCS 10552, pp. 12–19, 2017.
DOI: 10.1007/978-3-319-67534-3_2

of the stent. The IVUS images can be visualized in long-axis view, allowing a pullback-wise analysis and in short axis view allowing a frame-wise analysis (see Fig. 1(a and b)). The physician examines both views, identifying the presence of struts. The analysis of a single short-axis image sometimes is not sufficient for accurately assessing if struts are present. In most of ambiguous cases, the physician has to scroll the pullback back and forward, analyzing adjacent frames until the stent boundaries are detected.

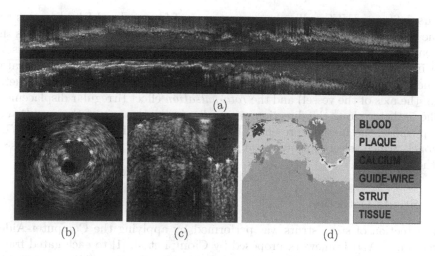

Fig. 1. Example of IVUS image in long axis view (a) and in short axis view (b, c). The IVUS image is represented in polar (b) and in cartesian (c) coordinates, along with the corresponding classification maps of the short-axis cartesian image (d). The detected struts are represented using a yellow (c) and black (d) star markers. The automatic stent shape is represented in dashed blue line. (Color figure online)

To date, all the approaches for automatic stent analysis in IVUS assume that the analyzed frame always contains a stent [1–5], and no strategies have been proposed so far for detecting the boundaries and the position of the stent along the pullback. Instead, this paper extends a previously published stent detection method [1] by identifying the presence (location and extension) of the stent along the pullback.

The pipeline of the framework requires the identification of the stable frames of the sequence using an image-based gating technique [6] and the reliable detection of stent struts [1]. Then, this paper introduces a measure of likelihood for a frame to contain a stent, which we call *stent presence*. A temporal series is obtained by computing such likelihood along the whole sequence. The mono-dimensional signal is modeled as a train of rectangular waves by using an iterative and multi-scale approximation of the signal to symbols using the SAX algorithm [7], which allows to obtain a robust binary representation of the presence of the stent in the pullback.

In order to extensively validate the proposed CAD system, we collected a set of 80 IVUS in-vivo sequences. The data sets includes about 700 IVUS images containing metallic stents.

2   Method

2.1   Gating

Let us define an IVUS pullback as a sequence of frames $I = \{f_i\}$ where i is the frame number of the sequence. In the proposed pipeline, we first pre-process the pullback by applying an image-based gating procedure. Gating is a necessary step in order to make the analysis robust to two kinds of artifacts generated by the heart beating: the *swinging* effect (repetitive oscillations of the catheter along the axis of the vessel) and the *roto-pulsation* effect (irregular displacement of the catheter along the direction perpendicular to the axis of the vessel). For this purpose, the method presented by Gatta et al. [6] is applied to the IVUS pullback, which selects a sequence of gated frames $G = \{f_{g_j}\}$ that are processed by the system.

2.2   Struts Detection

The detection of stent struts was performed by applying the Computer-Aided Detection (CAD) framework proposed by Ciompi et al. [1] to each gated frame independently. The method, provides a reliable identification of the stent struts, by contemporaneously considering the textural appearance of the stent and the vessel morphology. The CAD system uses the Multi-Scale Multi-Class Stacked Sequential Learning (M^{2}SSL) classification scheme to provide a comprehensive interpretation of the local structure of the vessel. In the classification problem, the class *Strut* is considered as one of the six considered classes (defined as Blood area, Plaque, Calcium, Guide-wire shadow, Strut and external Tissues). For semantic classification purposes, tailored features used for classification to the problem [8] are used.

For each pixel $p(x,y)$ of a gated IVUS image, a classification map M is obtained (see Fig. 1(c)). A curve approximating the stent shape S_{shape} is initially estimated considering vascular constrains and classification results. For each region of M labelled as stent ($M_{\{S\}}$), a strut candidate is considered. The selected struts $p_s(x,y)$ were selected among the candidates, considering both local *appearance* and distance with respect to the stent shape S_{shape}. Consequently false positives candidates were discarded, and the regions containing a selected strut struts $M^*_{\{S\}}$ are a subset of $M_{\{S\}}$.

2.3   Stent Presence Assessment

The frames of the pullback corresponding to the vessel positions where the stent begins and ends can be identified by analyzing the detected struts. We model the

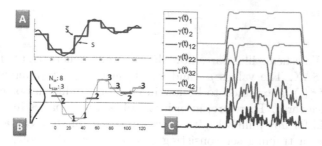

Fig. 2. Piecewise Aggregate Approximation of a generic signal (a) and quantization of $\gamma(t)$ after gaussian normalization (b). In (c) iterations of the SAX algorithm over an exemplar signal $\gamma(t)$ are illustrated.

presence of stent as a rectangular function $\sqcap(t)$, where the variable t indicates the spatial position in the pullback. We estimate the binary signal $\sqcap(t)$ by processing a real-valued signal $\gamma(t)$, which we define *stent presence*, corresponding to the frame-based likelihood of finding a stent in each frame of the IVUS sequence. The value of $\gamma(t)$ for each position t in the sequence is computed by considering both the number of struts and their area, thus negatively weights small struts areas of the images which have an high probability to be incorrect an detection. The function $\gamma(t)$ is defined as follows:

$$\gamma(t) = \sum_{p \in M^*_{\{S\}}} p|_{p_s \in M^*_{\{S\}}} \tag{1}$$

where $p_s \in M^*_{\{S\}}$ indicates the pixels of the IVUS frame labeled as *strut* containing an selected strut. An example of signal $\gamma(t)$ is depicted in Fig. 2(c).

The signal $\gamma(t)$ may contain several transitions between low and high amplitudes, due to the variability in the number of struts visible in consecutive frames and to suboptimal struts detection. For this reason, we filter the $\gamma(t)$ signal by considering its local statistics applying the SAX algorithm [7]. SAX is a symbolic representation algorithm that estimates a quantization of the time series based on global signal measurements and on local statistics of subsequent neighbor samples. Given the signal $\gamma(t)$ and a window size w, the algorithm calculates a Piecewise Aggregate Approximation (PAA) $\widehat{\gamma(t)}$, which is obtained by computing the local average values of $\gamma(t)$ over n_w segments w-wide. Each average value is then normalized over the signal $\gamma(t)$. The procedure firstly computes a vector $\overline{\gamma(t)} = (\overline{q}_1, ... \overline{q}_{n_w})$ where each of $\overline{q}_i$ is calculated as follows:

$$\overline{q}_i = \frac{1}{w} \sum_{j=w(i-1)+1}^{w \cdot i} q_j, \tag{2}$$

where $i, j \in \mathbb{N}$. Then, considering a Gaussian distribution of the samples, the quantified values $\widehat{q}_i$ are obtained by normalizing $\overline{q}_i$ by the mean μ_γ and standard deviation σ_γ of the signal $\gamma(t)$:

$$\widehat{q}_i = \frac{\overline{q}_i - \mu_\gamma}{\sigma_\gamma} \tag{3}$$

In Fig. 2(a, b) a scheme illustrates how the PPA of a generic signal is computed by applying SAX. The values μ_γ and σ_γ of each $\gamma(t)$ are different, since the amplitude of $\gamma(t)$ is expected to be low in case of a pullback not containing a stent, and vice-versa. Therefore, in order to obtain a global estimation of such variables valid for any pullbacks, it is necessary to estimate mean and standard deviation over a training set consisting of a representative collection of stent pullbacks.

The SAX algorithm is iterated N_{sax} times, until converging to flat intervals along the signal $\gamma(t)$. Figure 2(c) illustrates the iteration of the SAX algorithm over an exemplar signal $\gamma(t)$. The maximum iteration number N_{sax} is achieved when the difference between subsequent iterations of SAX is zero. The other parameters of the SAX algorithm is the number of quantized values assigned to the signal L_{sax}. The iterative SAX algorithm is described by the following equation:

$$\gamma(t)_{k+1} = SAX\left(\gamma(t)_k, \sigma_k^{train_{sax}}, \mu_k^{train_{sax}}, L^{train_{sax}}\right) \tag{4}$$

where $k \in 1..N_{sax}$ and $\sigma_k^{train_{sax}}$ and $\mu_k^{train_{sax}}$ are the mean and standard deviation computed on the training set at the iteration k, and the number of quantized values L_{sax} is a constant that has been optimized using the training set. When the SAX algorithm reaches the maximum iteration number N_{sax}, the binary signal indicating the stent presence of the stent is obtained as $\sqcap(t) = \gamma(t)_{N_{sax}} > \mu_{N_{sax}}^{train_{sax}}$.

3 Validation

3.1 Material

A set of 80 IVUS sequences containing a stent was collected. Roughly 50% of the frames contained a stent. The IVUS sequences were acquired using iLab echograph (Boston Scientific, Fremont, CA) with a 40 MHz catheter. The pullback speed was 0.5 mm/s.

Two experts (one clinician and one experienced researcher) manually annotated the beginning and the end of the stent in each sequence; more than one annotation per pullback was allowed when several stents were implanted in subsequent segments of the same artery.

3.2 Experiments on Stent Presence Assessment

The assessment of stent presence is based on the analysis of the monodimensional signal $\gamma(t)$. In order to evaluate the performance, the manual annotations of beginning and end of the stent were converted into binary signals $\gamma_{man}(t)$ indicating the presence of the stent in the pullback. Successively, the signals $\sqcap(t)$ indicating the segments of the pullback in which a stent is likely to be present, were compared against the sections indicated by the observers $\gamma_{man}(t)$. The performance were evaluated applying the algorithm to the sets $test_{met}$ and $test_{abs}$ and measures of *Precision (P), Recall (R), F-Measure (F),* and *Jaccard-index (J)* were considered.

In our experiments, we used the training set $train_{met}$ to estimate $\sigma_k^{train_{sax}}$, $\mu_k^{train_{sax}}$ and $L^{train_{sax}}$. The optimal number of quantized values assigned to the signal L_{sax} was chosen via cross-validation finding the value of $L_{sax} = 36$ as optimal.

Table 1. Quantitative evaluation the pullback analysis stage on both $test_{met}$ and $test_{abs}$ data-sets. For each data-set the performance of the automatic method versus each manual annotation are reported. Then the inter-observer variability is shown.

		Precision mean (std)	Recall mean (std)	F-measure mean (std)	Jaccard mean (std)
$test_{met}$	*auto* vs *obs-1*	85.4% (13.2%)	85.7% (7.7%)	84.8% (5.3%)	73.8% (13.7%)
	auto vs *obs-2*	89.5% (12.0%)	76.0% (10.6%)	80.7% (6.7%)	68.0% (13.8%)
	obs-1 vs *obs-2*	81.4% (11.3%)	98.8% (7.7%)	87.2% (7.8%)	80.7% (11.8%)

The quantitative results for the pullback-wise analysis is reported in Table 1. As IVUS is highly challenging to interpret, the two observers sometimes disagrees as shown Table 1. The precision approaches the inter-observer variability, while the recall is in general 10% lower than the results of the manual annotation. The obtained F-measure and the Jaccard measure of the automatic performance show satisfactory results when compared with manual annotations.

4   Results and Discussion

Examples of processed signals for the stent detection in IVUS frames are depicted in Fig. 3. In Fig. 3-(A1 and B1), both initial and final frame of the sequence are accurately identified. The result is not obvious since in (a) the amplitude of the signal $\gamma(t)$ is almost null in two sections of the pullback. However, the SAX algorithm allowed to detect the presence of stent, based on the statistics of the frames in the neighbourhood. On the other hand, in Fig. 3(A2), the central section of the pullback where $\gamma_{auto}(t)$ is almost null is correctly classified by the SAX algorithm as absence of stent. This is coherent with the manual annotation of the two observers, where two stents are labeled. In Fig. 3(B1 and B2), regions of high signal separated from the main stent have been identified as a secondary implanted stent. It might be noticed that this error happens only when strong spikes in the signal are present, for instance when a calcified plaque is mistaken for a deployed stent.

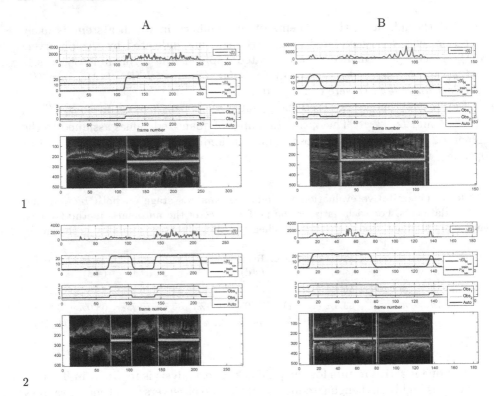

Fig. 3. Qualitative evaluation on $test_{met}$. The signal $\gamma(t)$ is illustrated in the first row, while in the second the result of the SAX quantization is reported. Finally in the third row, three binary signals representing the presence or the absence of the signal are compared: the first correspond to the automatic results, while the second and the third are the annotations of the two observers.

5   Conclusion

In this paper, a framework for the automatic identification of stent presence along the pullback (location and extension) has been presented. The analysis of the *stent presence* signal has been performed using the SAX algorithm with provides an unsupervised classification of the stent location in a fast and statistically robust fashion. The method has been implemented in Matlab and the computation time of the pullback analysis is about 4.1 s, one order of magnitude lower than the time required for detecting the stents [1] (33 s per pullback). Future work will be addressed towards validating the method with a larger data-set, including bio-absorbable stents.

Acknowledgments. This work was supported in part by the MICINN Grant TIN2015-66951-C2-1-R, SGR 1219, CERCA and ICREA Academia'2014.

References

1. Ciompi, F., Balocco, S., Rigla, J., Carrillo, X., Mauri, J., Radeva, P.: Computer-aided detection of intra-coronary stent in intravascular ultrasound sequences **43**(10), 5616–5625 (2016)
2. Canero, C., Pujol, O., Radeva, P., Toledo, R., Saludes, J., Gil, D., Villanueva, J., Mauri, J., Garcia, B., Gomez, J.: Optimal stent implantation: three-dimensional evaluation of the mutual position of stent and vessel via intracoronary echocardiography. In: Computers in Cardiology, pp. 261–264 (1999)
3. Dijkstra, J., Koning, G., Tuinenburg, J., Oemrawsingh, P., Reiber, J.: Automatic border detection in intravascular iltrasound images for quantitative measurements of the vessel, lumen and stent parameters. In: Computers in Cardiology 2001, vol. 28 (Cat. No. 01CH37287), vol. 1230, pp. 25–28 (2001)
4. Dijkstra, J., Koning, G., Tuinenburg, J.C., Oemrawsingh, P.V., Reiber, J.H.: Automatic stent border detection in intravascular ultrasound images. In: International Congress Series, vol. 1256, pp. 1111–1116. Elsevier (2003)
5. Rotger, D., Radeva, P., Bruining, N.: Automatic detection of bioabsorbable coronary stents in ivus images using a cascade of classifiers. IEEE Trans. Inform. Technol. Biomed. **14**, 535–537 (2010)
6. Gatta, C., Balocco, S., Ciompi, F., Hemetsberger, R., Leor, O.R., Radeva, P.: Real-time gating of IVUS sequences based on motion blur analysis: method and quantitative validation. In: Jiang, T., Navab, N., Pluim, J.P.W., Viergever, M.A. (eds.) MICCAI 2010. LNCS, vol. 6362, pp. 59–67. Springer, Heidelberg (2010). doi:10.1007/978-3-642-15745-5_8
7. Lin, J., Keogh, E., Wei, L., Lonardi, S.: Experiencing sax: a novel symbolic representation of time series. Data Min. Knowl. Disc. **15**, 107 (2007)
8. Ciompi, F., Pujol, O., Gatta, C., Alberti, M., Balocco, S., Carrillo, X., Mauri-Ferre, J., Radeva, P.: Holimab: a holistic approach for media-adventitia border detection in intravascular ultrasounds. Med. Image Anal. **16**, 1085–1100 (2012)

Robust Automatic Graph-Based Skeletonization of Hepatic Vascular Trees

R. Plantefève[1,2], S. Kadoury[1,2], A. Tang[2], and I. Peterlik[3,4(✉)]

[1] Ecole Polytechnique de Montrèal, Montreal, Canada
[2] CRCHUM, Montreal, Canada
[3] Inria, Strasbourg, France
[4] Institute of Computer Science, Masaryk University, Brno, Czech Republic
igor.peterlik@inria.fr

Abstract. The topologies of vascular trees embedded inside soft tissues carry important information which can be successfully exploited in the context of the computer-assisted planning and navigation. For example, topological matching of complete and/or partial hepatic trees provides important source of correspondences that can be employed straightforwardly by image registration algorithms. Therefore, robust and reliable extraction of vascular topologies from both pre- and intra-operative medical images is an important task performed in the context of surgical planning and navigation. In this paper, we propose an extension of an existing graph-based method where the vascular topology is constructed by computation of shortest paths in a minimum-cost spanning tree obtained from binary mask of the vascularization. We suppose that the binary mask is extracted from a 3D CT image using automatic segmentation and thus suffers from important artefacts and noise. When compared to the original algorithm, the proposed method (i) employs a new weighting measure which results in smoothing of extracted topology and (ii) introduces a set of tests based on various geometric criteria which are executed in order to detect and remove spurious branches. The method is evaluated on vascular trees extracted from abdominal contrast-enhanced CT scans and MR images. The method is quantitatively compared to the original version of the algorithm showing the importance of proposed modifications. Since the branch testing depends on parameters, the parametric study of the proposed method is presented in order to identify the optimal parametrization.

Keywords: Skeletonization · Segmentation · Computer-aided surgery · Hepatic vascular structures

1 Introduction

Liver cancer is the 7th most common cause of cancer death in Europe with around 62,200 deaths in 2012 [1]. In order to improve the success rate of interventional liver cancer treatment, several computer-aided approaches have been proposed for both intervention planning and navigation.

© Springer International Publishing AG 2017
M.J. Cardoso et al. (Eds.): CVII-STENT/LABELS 2017, LNCS 10552, pp. 20–28, 2017.
DOI: 10.1007/978-3-319-67534-3_3

The common factor of methods proposed to facilitate hepatic interventions remains the necessity of reliable and robust extraction and analysis of the hepatic vascular structures. The liver vascularization plays an important role in many aspects: the volume that is removed during the hepatectomy depends directly on the topology of the vascular network [2]. Similarly, the registration methods often rely on vascular landmarks [3]. Furthermore, accurate biomechanical models that are to be used in the augmented-reality applications must take into account the mechanical properties of the vascular trees [4,5].

While extremely important, the automatic robust analysis of liver vascularization remains a challenging problem. First, the liver displays a high inter-patient anatomic variability. Further, the acquisitions following the injection of a contrast agent, necessary for the pre-operative identification of vascular trees, often suffer from noise due to the respiratory motion which in turn deteriorates the quality of segmentation that is necessary for the extraction of the topological structure in the process known as skeletonization.

Several methods of skeletonization of vascular structures have been proposed in the literature. In [6], the thinning is applied to the binary mask to obtain the skeleton. Since the thinned structure remains a binary image, additional analysis is needed to extract the topological information. A skeletonization method is also proposed in [7], however, since the method works with surface meshes, it requires the extraction of such a mesh from the binary mask. In [8], another method based on Dijkstra minimum-cost spanning tree and which takes as input a binary mask is presented. In their paper, the authors test the method on phantom and clinical data acquired in neurosurgery. The same method is further extended and tested for airways tree skeletonization in [9].

In this paper, we focus on the skeletonization of vascular trees extracted from medical patient-specific data. We suppose that the skeletonization is performed on binary maps obtained by the automatic segmentation [10]. In this case, the resulting binary map typically suffers from artefacts, such as important surface bumps (see Fig. 1), making the skeletonization process very challenging. Therefore, we propose an extension of a graph-based method presented in [8] and [9]: first, we modify the algorithm to make is less sensitive w.r.t. the quality of the input data. Second, we propose a set of tests allowing for automatic removal of spurious or false branches relying on geometric criteria. The proposed skeletonization method is evaluated on 3 porcine and 32 human vascular trees and the results are compared to the original version of the algorithm. Moreover, a parametrization study is presented, showing the influence of method parameters on the quality of constructed skeleton.

2 Methods

2.1 Minimum-Cost Spanning Tree

The method based on the minimum-cost spanning tree [8] is applied directly to the binary map of the vascular structure which is converted into a weighted 3D graph where each voxel belonging to the segmented volume is represented

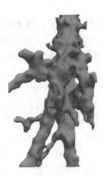

Fig. 1. Illustration of the automatically segmented binary map of hepatic vascularization.

by a weighted node. The method constructs the skeleton in two steps: First, the spanning tree is constructed iteratively starting from the root voxel. In the actual version of the algorithm, the root voxel is selected interactively in the area close to the root of the vascular tree. This is the only step of the method which currently requires manual intervention. Then, the edges between voxels are constructed recursively using a sorted heap: in each step, the head of the heap having the minimal weight is marked and all its unmarked neighbors are inserted into the heap. In [8], the sorting weight $w(v)$ of a voxel v is defined as $\frac{1}{r_b(v)}$, where $r_b(v)$ is the shortest distance of the voxel v from the boundary of the segmented vessel. We employ a modified definition the sorting weight $w(v) = w(u) + \frac{d(u,v)}{r_b(v)^k}$ where u is the voxel preceding v in the minimum-cost spanning tree, and $d(u,v)$ is the Euclidean distance between the voxels u and v. The metric $r_b(v)$ is pre-computed for each voxel of the input binary map. The modified definition of the heap-sorting weight makes the skeletonization process less sensitive to the bumps of the segmented vascular tree illustrated in Fig. 1. For each visited voxel, its distance from the tree root d_r is stored.

In the second phase of the method, the centerlines are extracted recursively from the spanning tree as in [8]:

- The 0-order path P_0 is constructed as the shortest path connecting the root and the voxel with the highest d_r in the graph, that is the voxel which is at the farest outlet from the root.
- Any n-order path P_n for $n > 0$ is extracted in three steps. First, an expansion step is performed so that for each voxel r of the path P_{n-1}, a set V_r of all voxels accessible throught the minimum-cost spanning tree from r is constructed. V_r is the set of all voxels that are linked to r and not belonging to P_{n-1}. Second, a voxel $t \in V_v$ having the maximum value d_r is found. Finally, the new path is constructed as the shortest path from r to t, denoted as (r, t).

2.2 Typical Artefacts of Graph-Based Skeletonization

The algorithm of the centerline extraction performs well on the synthetic data as well as real data where the vascular structures are represented by smooth and well-formed pipes. However, when applied to real data obtained using automatic segmentation of hepatic veins, artefacts appear resulting in false branches, i. e., redundant bifurcations.

First, directly during the construction of a path (r, t), it is verified that none of the voxels except r is already included in a path constructed before, i. e. there is no collision between the new path and any previously constructed path. While such situation should not happen due to the properties of the spanning tree, exceptions might occur, i. e. when holes or plate-shaped structures are present in the input binary mask.

The second type of artefacts is introduced by scenarios depicted in Fig. 2: for the sake of reference, we divide the scenarios in *T-shapes* (Fig. 2a, b) and *V-shapes* (Fig. 2c, d). In the case of T-shapes, the bumps (a) created by the automatic segmentation are difficult to distinguish from real branches (b). In the case of V-shapes, the problematic scenarios occur when a redundant centerline appears in the graph due to the vessel thickening (c). While from the anatomical point of view, such phenomenon is improbable, it is not rare in binary masks produced by the automatic segmentation.

2.3 Filtering of Spurious Branches

In order to prevent the extraction of false branches, we propose to filter the branches directly during the extraction of paths based on several criteria. First, let us denote R the geometrical position in Cartesian coordinates of the branch candidate root voxel r, T the position of its tip voxel t and finally C the position of voxel c on the parent branch which has the lowest Euclidean distance from T. In the following description of the algorithm, we always refer to Fig. 2.

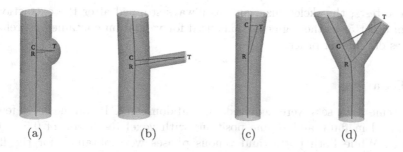

(a)   (b)   (c)   (d)

Fig. 2. Different scenarios occurring during skeletonization of automatically segmented vessels. T-shape scenarios: (a) false path due to the surface bump, (b) correct branch. V-shape scenarios: (c) false path due to the vessel thickening, (d) correct branch: the background voxels shown in red. (Color figure online)

Table 1. Evaluation of the graph-based algorithm on the swine hepatic tree.

	# path candidates	# accepted			# rejected			
		all	T-shape(b)	V-shape(d)	all	collision	T-shape(a)	V-shape(c)
Flank hepatic	5797	259	62	197	5538	530	5006	2
Flank portal	2064	57	12	45	2007	90	1916	1
Supine hepatic	4027	144	95	49	3883	249	3632	2

1. If $|TR| < L_{\text{thr}} d_b(r)$, the branch candidate is rejected. Here, the $d_b(r)$ is distance from boundary of the root voxel r and L_{thr} is a parameter, *length threshold*. This parameter is a unitless quantity which determines the relative ratio between a child branch having an acceptable length and the thickness of the parent branch. The goal of this step is to eliminate the short false branches produced either inside the tube of the parent branch or due to the bumps (a).
2. In the next step, the correct V-shapes are identified (d). In this case, there exist voxels on the line CT (connecting the voxels c and t) located outside of the binary mask. Such *background voxels* guarantee that path is located in a child branch which is correctly detached from the parent branch. Therefore, in this step, the path candidate for which such voxels exist is directly accepted as a new path and the algorithm proceeds with extraction of another path.
3. The branch candidate that made it to this step is sufficiently long but has no background voxel. Therefore, it corresponds either to valid T-shape (b) or invalid V-Shape (c). In order to distinguish the two cases, we introduce the second parameter, *angle threshold* A_{thr}. The path candidate is accepted if the angle $\angle CRT > A_{\text{thr}}$, otherwise, it is rejected.

The algorithm stops when no new branches are added in the actual order.

3   Results

In all the tests, the skeletonization was always stopped after the extraction of paths of order 5, as the segmentations used for validation contained no reliable branches of a higher order.

3.1   Data

The porcine data sets were acquired from abdominal CT volumes of a female pig scanned in flank and supine positions with voxel resolution of $0.5 \times 0.5 \times 0.5$ mm^3. While both portal and venous phases were obtained for the flank position, only the venous phase was available for the supine configuration, thus resulting in three data sets. The human data sets were acquired from abdominal CT and MR volume with voxel resolution of $0.68 \times 0.68 \times 2.0$ mm^3 and $1.0 \times 1.0 \times 2.5$ mm^3, respectively. A retrospective cohort of fifteen patients (4 women, 11 men) that received a bi-phasic magnetic resonance angiography (MRA) and computed tomography angiography (CTA) on the same day were included in this study. The MRA images were acquired on the Achieva 3T scanner (Philips Healthcare, Best, The Netherlands) using a 3D mDIXON sequence and on the Discovery MR450 scanner (GE medical Systems, Milwaukee,WI,USA) using the 3D LAVA sequence. CTA images were acquired using the helical mode on the Brillance 64 scanner (Philips Healthcare, Best, The Netherlands) and the Bright-Speed system (GE Medical Systems, Milwaukee, WI, USA). Vascular structures were segmented in each data set using an automatic method [10].

3.2 Evaluation of the Skeletonization

The graph-based skeletonization is evaluated in Table 1 for each vascular tree. First, a large number of path candidates is extracted from the spanning tree. The most significant reduction of candidates happens due to the insufficient length of the candidate branch: more than 85% of candidates are false child branches, i. e. too short when compared to the thickness of the parent branch. Less than 10% of candidates are removed because of crossing with other branches (potential cycles). Finally, less then 5% of candidates are accepted as new paths: majority of them are accepted as *V-shape* vessels.

3.3 Method Parametrization

As introduced in Sect. 2.3, the graph-based skeletonization method requires two parameters: the length threshold L_{thr} and the parent–child angle threshold A_{thr}. As for the latter, very low sensitivity was observed w.r.t. this parameter: only from 1 to 2 false *V-shape* candidates appeared during the extraction and were eliminated by setting the threshold to 20°. This observation confirms that the construction of the spanning tree already prevents the formation false *V-shape* paths.

In contrast, the value of L_{thr} influences the filtering significantly. Intuitively, a logical choice for this parameter is 1; it should be sufficient to filter all the candidates having the length shorter that the thickness of the parent branch. However, this assumption is not valid when bumps are present in the input data (Fig. 2). The size of the bumps can make it difficult to distinguish them from short real branches; see Fig. 1 showing a sample of the real data used for testing.

In order to study the influence of L_{thr} on the skeletonization of the vascular trees, we have performed a scaling of the parameter starting from 1.0 to 2.0;

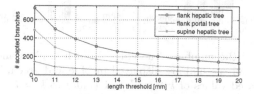

Fig. 3. Number of accepted branches w.r.t. the length threshold.

the result is presented in Fig. 3. The plot shows that the number of accepted branches decreases rapidly from 1.0 to 1.4; then, the decreasing slope becomes less steep. Although it is not possible to specify the cut-off value which would allow for reliable filtering of the false branches while keeping the real ones, we propose using the value 1.4 as the threshold. The values in Table 1 have been obtained with this parameter.

3.4   Original vs. Modified Skeletonization Method

In order to assess the method, we have compared the proposed approach to the method presented in [8]. We used 32 segmentations performed using the ITK-Snap semi-automatic segmentation algorithm based on active contour (Snakes, [11]) on computed tomography and magnetic resonance images. The segmentations corresponds either to human hepatic and splenic arteries or to the human hepatic portal vascular system.

The best accuracy computed as the number of accepted branches, i. e. the value for which the error in the branch number is minimal, is obtained for both algorithms with $L_{thr} = 2.5$ regardless the values of the other parameters. Thus, this value was used for the comparison of the two methods. With higher values true branches are rejected as outliers. Figure 4 shows the number of accepted branches by the two algorithms versus the real number of branches determined manually by an expert. The consistency of the branches were checked manually for all datasets. The evaluation shows that the number of branches extracted with the original algorithm proposed by Verscheure is slightly superior when compared to the values obtained by our algorithm. Most of the time, a false branch detected by Verscheure's algorithm runs in parallel to another branch (see Fig. 5). Interestingly, even without an angle threshold, our modified method

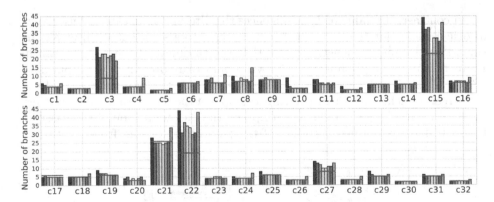

Fig. 4. Comparison of the number of accepted branches; cN stands for the case N. The results given by our method are displayed in blue and green. The color gradient corresponds to increased values of k from $k = 1$ (blue) to $k = 7$ (green). The results of Verscheure's algorithm are displayed in yellow. The red horizontal line depicts the number of real branches for each case. (Color figure online)

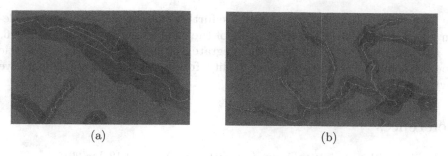

(a)   (b)

Fig. 5. False branches running parrallel to another branch. Results obtained by Verscheure's algorithm.

produces on average 3 times less parallel branches when compared to the original method. The failing cases are encountered for very noisy segmentation maps for which the bumps are too large for the false branches to be filtered out by the length threshold. Another important source of differences between the two algorithms is given by false loops which occur when distance between distinct branches remains under the resolution of the segmented image, leading to topological errors.

The shape of the extracted centerlines depend also on the exponent k employed in the definition of the heap-sorting weight $w(v) = w(u) + \frac{d(u,v)}{r_b(v)^k}$: For $k \leq 3$, the centerlines tend to be rather straight and do not follow the shape of the vessel properly. This is particularly obvious for tortuous vessels such as the splenic arteries. Therefore, we recommend to use $k > 3$.

4 Conclusions

In this paper, we have presented a method of automatic skeletonization of vascular trees. The algorithm was assessed on binary masks automatically segmented from abdominal CT scans of a porcine liver. It was shown that it is possible to select parametrization to suppress the false branches introduced by the noise in

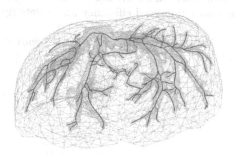

Fig. 6. Complete skeleton of the hepatic tree in porcine liver.

the input data. In the actual case, we have further smoothed the extracted skeleton using cubic splines. The illustration of the complete tree is shown in Fig. 6.

In the future work, we plan to integrate the algorithm to an automatic pipeline employed in an augmented-reality framework for the intra-operative navigation in hepatic surgery.

References

1. World health organization. http://www.who.int. Accessed 12 Jun 2015
2. Mise, Y., Tani, K., Aoki, T., Sakamoto, Y., Hasegawa, K., Sugawara, Y., Kokudo, N.: Virtual liver resection: computer-assisted operation planning using a three-dimensional liver representation. J. Hepato-Biliary-Pancreat. Sci. **20**(2), 157–164 (2013)
3. Ambrosini, P., Ruijters, D., Niessen, W.J., Moelker, A., van Walsum, T.: Continuous roadmapping in liver tace procedures using 2D-3D catheter-based registration. Int. J. Comput. Assist. Radiol. Surg. **10**(9), 1357–1370 (2015)
4. Peterlík, I., Duriez, C., Cotin, S.: Modeling and real-time simulation of a vascularized liver tissue. In: Medical Image Computing and Computer-Assisted Intervention-MICCAI 2012. Springer 50–57 (2012)
5. Plantefève, R., Peterlik, I., Haouchine, N., Cotin, S.: Patient-specific biomechanical modeling for guidance during minimally-invasive hepatic surgery. Ann. Biomed. Eng. **44**(1), 139–153 (2016)
6. Lee, T.C., Kashyap, R.L., Chu, C.N.: Building skeleton models via 3-D medial surface axis thinning algorithms. CVGIP. Graph. Models Image Process. **56**(6), 462–478 (1994)
7. Piccinelli, M., Veneziani, A., Steinman, D.A., Remuzzi, A., Antiga, L.: A framework for geometric analysis of vascular structures: application to cerebral aneurysms. IEEE Trans. Med. Imaging **28**(8), 1141–1155 (2009)
8. Verscheure, L., Peyrodie, L., Dewalle, A.S., Reyns, N., Betrouni, N., Mordon, S., Vermandel, M.: Three-dimensional skeletonization and symbolic description in vascular imaging: preliminary results. Int. J. Comput. Assist. Radiol. Surg. **8**(2), 233–246 (2013)
9. Valencia, L.F., Pinzón, A.M., Richard, J.C., Hoyos, M.H., Orkisz, M.: Simultaneous skeletonization and graph description of airway trees in 3D CT images. In: XXVème Colloque GRETSI (2015)
10. Yushkevich, P.A., et al.: User-guided 3D active contour segmentation of anatomical structures: significantly improved efficiency and reliability. Neuroimage **31**(3), 1116–1128 (2006)
11. Kass, M., Witkin, A., Terzopoulos, D.: Snakes: active contour models. Int. J. Comput. Vision **1**(4), 321–331 (1988)

DCNN-Based Automatic Segmentation and Quantification of Aortic Thrombus Volume: Influence of the Training Approach

Karen López-Linares[1,2,4](✉), Luis Kabongo[1,4], Nerea Lete[1,4],
Gregory Maclair[1,4], Mario Ceresa[2], Ainhoa García-Familiar[3], Iván Macía[1,4],
and Miguel Ángel González Ballester[2,5]

[1] Vicomtech-IK4 Foundation, San Sebastián, Spain
klopez@vicomtech.org
[2] Universitat Pompeu Fabra, Barcelona, Spain
[3] Hospital Universitario Donostia, San Sebastián, Spain
[4] Biodonostia Health Research Institute, San Sebastián, Spain
[5] ICREA, Barcelona, Spain

Abstract. Computerized Tomography Angiography (CTA) based assessment of Abdominal Aortic Aneurysms (AAA) treated with Endovascular Aneurysm Repair (EVAR) is essential during follow-up to evaluate the progress of the patient along time, comparing it to the pre-operative situation, and to detect complications. In this context, accurate assessment of the aneurysm or thrombus volume pre- and post-operatively is required. However, a quantifiable and trustworthy evaluation is hindered by the lack of automatic, robust and reproducible thrombus segmentation algorithms. We propose an automatic pipeline for thrombus volume assessment, starting from its segmentation based on a Deep Convolutional Neural Network (DCNN) both pre-operatively and post-operatively. The aim is to investigate several training approaches to evaluate their influence in the thrombus volume characterization.

Keywords: AAA · EVAR · Thrombus · Segmentation · DCNN · Volume

1 Introduction

An abdominal aortic aneurysm (AAA) is a focal dilation of the aorta that exceeds its normal diameter in more than 50%. If not treated, it tends to grow and may rupture, with a high mortality rate [1]. Lately, AAA treatment has shifted from open surgery to a minimally invasive alternative, known as Endovascular Aneurysm Repair (EVAR) [2]. This technique consists in the transfemoral insertion and deployment of a stent using a catheter. Although better peri-operative outcomes are achieved, long-term studies show similar mortality rates between patients treated with EVAR and patients treated with open surgery [3]. This is due to the appearance of EVAR related complications, known as endoleaks,

© Springer International Publishing AG 2017
M.J. Cardoso et al. (Eds.): CVII-STENT/LABELS 2017, LNCS 10552, pp. 29–38, 2017.
DOI: 10.1007/978-3-319-67534-3_4

which translate into a recurrent blood-flow into the thrombus area that causes its continuous growing, with the associated rupture risk and possible reintervention. Thus, post-operative surveillance is required to evaluate changes and detect possible complications, for which Computed Tomography Angiography (CTA) is the preferred imaging modality. This follow-up is traditionally based on the observation of CTA scans at different times and the manual measurement of the maximum aneurysm diameter, although AAA volume has been reported as a better predictor of the disease progression [4]. In [5], a fully-automatic thrombus segmentation approach based on a Deep Convolutional Neural Network (DCNN) was proposed, specifically designed for post-operative thrombus segmentation. Our aim is to extend that work by providing segmentation for both pre-operative and post-operative scenarios and to provide a full pipeline for thrombus volume assessment, investigating the influence of network training strategies in the automatic segmentation quality and volume quantification.

2   State-of-the-art

Historically, aneurysm size, measured through its largest diameter, has been the most commonly employed rupture risk indicator. This evaluation is done both pre-operatively, to determine if an intervention is required, and post-operatively, to assess the patient's progression. Thrombus volume seems to be a better rupture risk indicator [4], but it is hardly used in the clinical practice due to the lack of automatic thrombus segmentation methods. The thrombus appears as a non-contrasted structure in the CTA, its shape varies and its borders are fuzzy, which makes it difficult to develop robust automatic segmentation approaches. Thus, the subsequent precise and automatic thrombus characterization is unfeasible.

Currently there are only few dedicated software that provide assistance to EVAR-treated aneurysm follow-up: VesselIQ Xpress (GE) [6] and Vitrea Imaging (Toshiba) [7] allow the semi-automatic segmentation and volume quantification of the thrombus. Hence, recent research work aims at obtaining a robust, automatic thrombus segmentation algorithm easily applicable in the clinical practice. Traditionally proposed methods combine intensity information with shape constraints to minimize a certain energy function [8–10]. Machine learning approaches have also been proposed [11], as well as radial model methods [12]. In [13] a deformable model-based approximation was introduced and recently another deformable model approximation, validated in a large number of pre-operative and post-operative datasets has been presented in [14]. However, these algorithms require user interaction and/or prior lumen segmentation along with centerline extraction and their performance highly depends on multiple parameter tuning, affecting their robustness and clinical applicability.

Lately, DCNNs have gained attention in the scientific community for solving complex segmentation tasks, surpassing the previous state-of-the-art performance in many problems. In [15] a novel and automatic patch-based approach to pre-operative AAA region detection and segmentation is described, based on Deep Belief Networks (DBN). Comparison with ground truth segmentation was not provided. In [5], a DCNN for automatic post-operative thrombus segmentation and evaluation was presented. Our goal is to extend that work by providing pre-operative and post-operative AAA segmentation and volume quantification, training the network with more datasets and evaluating the influence of the training approximation in the subsequent thrombus volume measurement.

3   Methods

We propose an automatic approach to thrombus segmentation and volume quantification. Segmentation is based on a DCNN specifically designed to segment the thrombus in post-operative datasets, initially presented in [5]. The network is based on Fully Convolutional Networks [16] and Holistically-Nested Edge Detection network [17] and combines low-level features with coarser representations that ensure the smooth contour of the thrombus is kept. To evaluate the influence of the training strategy in the segmentation and volume quantification results, we carry out three experiments: first we train and test the network with mixed pre-operative and post-operative datasets; then, a separate training approach using only pre-operative or only post-operative data is included to compare the results and draw conclusions. Since the number of annotated quality data is limited, we train in a 2D slice-by-slice manner. Training in 2D provides advantages regarding speed, lower memory consumption and the ability to use pretrained networks and fine-tuning. These advantages are leveraged and the 3D coherence of the output binary segmentation is provided in a subsequent post-processing step. Finally, segmentation quality is evaluated by comparison with manually delineated ground truth segmentations. Thrombus volume is computed from the ground truth segmentation and the post-processed automatic segmentation to check the ability of the proposed approach to characterize the thrombus. A visual representation of these steps is shown in Fig. 1. Each step is further explained in the following subsections.

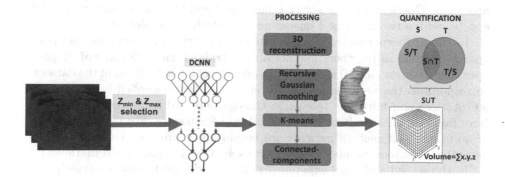

Fig. 1. Pipeline for automatic thrombus segmentation and volume quantification.

3.1 Abdominal Aortic Aneurysm Datasets

A total of 38 contrast-enhanced CTA datasets from different patients that present infrarenal aneurysms were employed for our experiments. 20 of them are post-operative datasets, while 18 of them correspond to pre-operative scans. These datasets have been obtained with scanners of different manufacturers and have a spatial resolution ranging from 0.725 to 0.977 in x and y, and 0.625-1 in z. They also have varying contrast agent doses. The patient is always located in supine position and the CTA starts around the diaphragm and expands to the iliac crest. The data have been divided into training and testing sets. Training data consists in 20 datasets, 11 post-operative and 9 pre-operative. Testing data is composed of 18 datasets, 9 post-operative and 9 pre-operative. None of the datasets correspond to the same patient. We did not discard datasets of patients with outlying characteristics, so the variability in the data is relatively large in terms of thrombus size and shape or noise. In the post-operative datasets of patients with a favorable evolution, endotension cases and datasets where a leak is visible have been included. For all the patients manually obtained segmentations are available and used as ground truths for the current study. Note that the number of pixels corresponding to the thrombus is much smaller than the number of pixels corresponding to background, with a mean ratio of approximately 1:8.

3.2 Experimental Setup: Thrombus Segmentation

As mentioned above, thrombus segmentation is based on a DCNN network, trained slice-by-slice. Figure 2 is a visual representation of the network architecture. Our goal is to investigate the influence of the training approach by performing three experiments. In the three of them, we train the same network architecture, with the same hyperparameters and try to minimize the Softmax loss, which reduces the influence of extreme values or outliers in the data and provides the probability of each pixel corresponding to a certain class. Learning rate is set 10e-3, with a step down policy of 33% and gamma equal to 0.1. The Stochastic Gradient Descent solver is employed and training is done during 100 epochs, with a batch size of 4 images and no batch accumulation.

In the first experiment, we train our network with pre-operative and post-operative data, all together. The network is trained with 2D slices of 11 post-operative datasets and 2D slices of 9 pre-operative datasets. None of the datasets correspond to the same patient. Data augmentation is applied in the form of 90 rotations and mirroring to enlarge the datasets and to prevent the network from failing if a rotated dataset is introduced for testing. For testing, datasets of additional different 18 patients are employed, 9 pre-operative and 9 post-operative. The total number of slices for each stage is summarized in Table 1.

In the second and third experiments, 2 networks are trained separately, one only with pre-operative data, the other one just with post-operative. For the pre-operative, 9 pre-operative datasets are used for training and validation, and 9 different datasets are saved for testing purposes. These datasets are identical to those of the first experiment, and the same data augmentation is applied. Testing is done on slices of patients not included in the training phase, as in the first experiment. In the third experiment, corresponding to the post-operative data, the same approximation is followed. The 11 post-operative datasets used for training on the first experiment are utilized to train this network, and the same 9 post-operative datasets are employed for testing. Data augmentation is also equally applied. Table 1 summarizes the data for these experiments.

Table 1. Training, validation and testing slices used in each experiment.

	Experiment 1	Experiment 2	Experiment 3
Train	4380	1835	2545
Validation	772	323	449
Testing	2878	1447	1431

3.3 Post-processing and Quantification

The output provided by the DCNN are 2D probability maps, where each intensity value is the probability of that pixel being thrombus or not. Thus, an automatic processing of these maps is included as the last step to obtain the 3D binary mask segmentation. First, we reconstruct the 3D prediction map volume and apply Gaussian filtering in the z-direction to ensure some continuity in this direction. We set the sigma value to $\sigma = 2 * Spacing_z$. Then, K-means clustering of the 3D probability map is employed, where the number of clusters is fixed to 6, experimentally. The output cluster image is filtered and binarized, by removing the class with the lowest probability of being thrombus. A subsequent connected component analysis is used to keep the largest object, which in our experiments always corresponds to the thrombus. The Volume is measured based on the Divergence Theorem Algorithm (DTA), by estimating the volume of the thrombus from its point-list, as explained in [18]. Finally, a comparison between the automatic thrombus binary segmentation (source, S) and the expert delineated ground truth (target, T) is included to evaluate segmentation quality in terms of total overlap, Dice coefficient, false negative rate (FN) and false positive rate (FP), as proposed in [19]. The volume difference between both segmentations is also included.

$Total\ overlap\ for\ thrombus\ region\ (r): |\ S_r \cap T_r\ |\ /\ |\ T_r\ |$
$Dice\ coefficient\ for\ thrombus\ region\ (r):\ 2\ |\ S_r \cap T_r\ |\ /(|\ S_r\ |\ +\ |\ T_r\ |)$
$False\ negative\ error\ for\ thrombus\ region\ (r): |\ T_r/S_r\ |\ /\ |\ T_r\ |$
$False\ positive\ error\ for\ thrombus\ region\ (r): |\ S_r/T_r\ |\ /\ |\ S_r\ |$
$Volume\ difference: |\ V_T - V_S\ |\ /V_T$

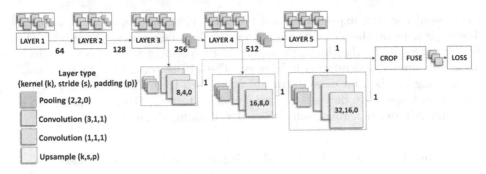

Fig. 2. Deep convolutional neural network architecture for thrombus segmentation.

4   Results

Table 2 summarizes the results for the first experiment, where the network is trained and tested both with pre-operative and post-operative data. The mean Dice similarity coefficient is 81.4%, being this coefficient higher in the post-operative than in the pre-operative. Since the number of pre-operative slices is smaller than the number of post-operative slices and the network was initially designed for the post-operative scenario, a reduction in the accuracy in the pre-operative could be expected. This also impacts the volume difference between the automatically segmented thrombus and the ground truth, being this difference larger in the pre-operative than in the post-operative. The mean volume difference is 12.8%, where the over-estimation of the volume is of 10.9% and the sub-estimation is of 13.9%. Sub-estimation occurs in the double of cases where over-estimation occurs. Qualitative results of this experiment are shown in Fig. 3.

In the second and third experiments, we trained the same network but only with pre-operative or post-operative data. Results are reported in Table 2. In the pre-operative, contrary to our initial hypothesis that an improvement should be observed when training two networks separately, a reduction in the Dice coefficient and an increase of the volume difference is obtained compared to the first experiment. We attribute these results to the reduction in the number of training samples, being only slices extracted from 9 different datasets. Hence, the ability of the network to generalize diminishes. When testing, the variability in the aneurysm shape affects more notably the segmentation quality, and the results for one testing dataset have a stronger impact on the global mean. The worst result for a pre-operative dataset corresponds to the case depicted in Fig. 4, where there is contrasted blood inside the aneurysm area. Probably, the network does not expect to find high-contrasted areas that are not lumen, stent or calcifications, which always set the limits for the segmentation, and thus, it understands that there is a border in this contrasted area and sub-segments the aneurysm; without this dataset the mean Dice coefficient would be equal to 72.8% and the volume difference would be 14%, which approximates to the results of the first experiment, but with half the number of training images.

Table 2. Testing results for the three experiments: 1) the network is trained and tested both with pre-operative and post-operative data, 2) the network is trained only with pre-operative data, 3) only post-operative data is employed.

Experiment		Total overlap	Dice	FN	FP	Volume difference
1	Pre	0.784 ± 0.127	0.790 ± 0.102	0.216 ± 0.127	0.193 ± 0.103	0.134 ± 0.093
	Post	0.817 ± 0.066	0.837 ± 0.062	0.183 ± 0.066	0.133 ± 0.095	0.121 ± 0.081
	Mean	0.801 ± 0.103	0.814 ± 0.087	0.199 ± 0.103	0.163 ± 0.103	0.128 ± 0.088
2	Pre	0.616 ± 0.171	0.697 ± 0.132	0.384 ± 0.171	0.154 ± 0.076	0.265 ± 0.220
3	Post	0.886 ± 0.058	0.855 ± 0.065	0.134 ± 0.058	0.152 ± 0.087	0.086 ± 0.080

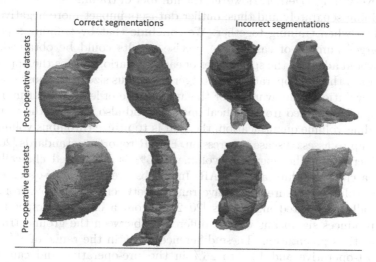

Fig. 3. Qualilative segmentation results of the first experiment. The manual ground truth is shown in green and the automatic segmentation in yellow. (Color figure online)

With respect to the third experiment, related to the post-operative, an increase of the Dice coefficient and a decrease on the volume difference is observed, which agrees with our hypothesis that by training both scenarios separately, better results can be expected. A 33.9% improvement in the volume difference is achieved, although only half the number of training images have been utilized.

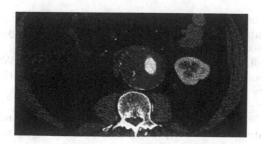

Fig. 4. Incorrect pre-operative AAA segmentation due to contrasted blood inside it.

5 Conclusions

In this paper, we have investigated the influence of the DCNN training strategy in the automatic segmentation and quantification of the AAA volume. Three experiments have been performed: first, the network has been trained and tested with both pre- and post-operative datasets; then, two networks have been trained separately, only with pre- or post-operative data. The same training and testing datasets are used for all the experiments, which correspond to different patients. The results showed that by training separately for the pre-operative and the post-operative scenarios, similar or even better results could be obtained compared to training everything together. However, the number of training samples is smaller when training separately and thus, outlier datasets impact more negatively the results than when training together. We conclude that by training separately with a larger number of cases more precise results could be obtained. Each network would adapt to the specificities of each scenario, such as the appearance of the stent in the post-operative, the bigger thrombus size in the post-operative when the evolution is unfavorable or the appearance of leaks. Fine-tuning from network weights learned from medical images could also improve the results.

Regarding volume quantification, the goal is to utilize thrombus volume during follow-up to assess disease progression. EVAR reporting standards [20] state that an increase in the aneurysm volume of 5% is considered clinically relevant and a clinical failure after EVAR. Intra-observer and inter-observer variability for volume measurements have ranged between 3% and 5% from semi-automatically segmented aneurysms [20–22]. From a clinical perspective, our pipeline produces significant volume differences between the ground truth and the automatic segmentation. These differences vary in the range of 8% to 12% in the post-operative and 13% to 26% in the pre-operative and can equally correspond to over-estimation or sub-estimation of the volume. The automatic segmentation results are reasonably good, but the measured volume values still need to be refined to be directly applicable in the clinical practice for quantitative progression assessment. Future work aims at reducing the volume difference between ground truth and automatically segmented thrombus, by adapting our method to that purpose and analyzing the volume quantification results with more data.

References

1. Pearce, W.H., Zarins, C.K., Bacharach, J.M.: Atherosclerotic peripheral vascular disease symposium II: controversies in abdominal aortic aneurysm repair. Circulation 118(25), 2860–2863 (2008)
2. Moll, F.L., Powell, J.T., Fraedrich, G., Verzini, F., Haulon, S., Waltham, M., Ricco, J.B.: Management of abdominal aortic aneurysms clinical practice guidelines of the European society for vascular surgery. Eur. J. Vasc. Endovasc. Surg. 41(1), 1–58 (2011)
3. Stather, P.W., Sidloff, D., Dattani, N.: Systematic review and meta-analysis of the early and late outcomes of open and endovascular repair of abdominal aortic aneurysm. J. Vasc. Surg. 58(4), 1142 (2013)

4. Renapurkar, R.D., Setser, R.M., O'Donnell, T.P., Egger, J., Lieber, M.L., Desai, M.Y., Stillman, A.E., Schoenhagen, P., Flamm, S.D.: Aortic volume as an indicator of disease progression in patients with untreated infrarenal abdominal aneurysm. Eur. J. Radiol. **81**(2), 87–93 (2012)
5. López-Linares, K., Aranjuelo, N., Kabongo, L., Maclair, G., Lete, N., Leskovsky, P., Garca-Familiar, A., Macía, I., González Ballester, M.A.: Fully automatic segmentation of abdominal aortic thrombus in post-operative CTA images using deep convolutional neural networks. Proc. Int. J. CARS **12**(1), 29–30 (2017)
6. http://www3.gehealthcare.com/en/products/categories/advanced_visualization/applications/autobone_and_vesseliq_xpress
7. https://www.vitalimages.com/clinicalapplications/tabs/ct-endovascular-stent-planning
8. Duquette, A.A., Jodoin, P.M., Bouchot, O., Lalande, A.: 3D segmentation of abdominal aorta from CT-scan and MR images. Comput. Med. Imaging Graph. **36**(4), 294–303 (2012)
9. Egger, J., Freisleben, B., Setser, R., Renapuraar, R., Biermann, C., ODonnell, T.: Aorta segmentation for stent simulation. In: MICCAI Workshop on Cardiovascular Interventional Imaging and Biophysical Modelling, p. 10 (2009)
10. Freiman, M., Esses, S.J., Joskowicz, L., Sosna, J.: An iterative model-constrained graph-cut algorithm for abdominal aortic aneurysm thrombus segmentation. In: IEEE International Symposium on Biomedical Imaging: From Nano to Macro, pp. 672–675 (2010)
11. Maiora, J., Ayerdi, B., Graña, M.: Random forest active learning for AAA thrombus segmentation in computed tomography angiography images. Neurocomputing **126**, 71–77 (2014)
12. Macía, I., Legarreta, J.H., Paloc, C., Graña, M., Maiora, J., García, G., Blas, M.: Segmentation of abdominal aortic aneurysms in CT images using a radial model approach. In: Corchado, E., Yin, H. (eds.) IDEAL 2009. LNCS, vol. 5788, pp. 664–671. Springer, Heidelberg (2009). doi:10.1007/978-3-642-04394-9_81
13. Demirci, S., Lejeune, G., Navab, N.: Hybrid deformable model for aneurysm segmentation. In: IEEE International Symposium on Biomedical Imaging: From Nano to Macro, pp. 33–36 (2009)
14. Lalys, F., Yan, V., Kaladji, A., Lucas, A., Esneault, S.: Generic thrombus segmentation from pre- and post-operative CTA. Int. J. Comput. Assist. Radiol. Surg. **12**(9), 1501–1510 (2017)
15. Hong, H., Sheikh, U.: Automatic detection, segmentation and classification of abdominal aortic aneurysm using deep learning. In: 2016 IEEE 12th International Colloquium on Signal Process Its Application, pp. 242–246 (2016)
16. Long, J., Shelhamer, E., Darrell, T.: Fully convolutional networks for semantic segmentation. In: IEEE Conference on Computer Vision and Pattern Recognition, pp. 3431–3440 (2015)
17. Xie, S., Tu, Z.: Holistically-nested edge detection. CoRR abs/1504.06375 (2015)
18. Alyassin, A.M., Lancaster, J.L., Downs, J.H., Fox, P.T.: Evaluation of new algorithms for the interactive measurement of surface area and volume. Med Phys. **21**(6), 741–752 (1994)
19. Tustison, N., Gee, J.: Introducing dice, jaccard, and other label overlap measures to ITK. Insight J. (2009)
20. Chaikof, E., Blankensteijn, J., Harris, P., White, G., Zarins, C., et al.: Reporting standards for endovascular aortic aneurysm repair. J. Vasc. Surg. **35**(5), 1048–1060 (2002)

21. Parr, A., Jayaratne, C., Buttner, P., Golledge, J.: Comparison of volume and diameter measurement in assessing small abdominal aortic aneurysm expansion examined using computed tomographic angiography. Eur. J. Radiol. **79**(1), 42–47 (2011)
22. van Prehn, J., van der Wal, M.B., Vincken, K., Bartels, L.W., Moll, F.L., van Herwaarden, J.A.: Intra- and interobserver variability of aortic aneurysm volume measurement with fast CTA postprocessing software. J. Endovasc. Ther. **15**(5), 504–510 (2008)

Vascular Segmentation in TOF MRA Images of the Brain Using a Deep Convolutional Neural Network

Renzo Phellan[1]([⊠]), Alan Peixinho[2], Alexandre Falcão[2], and Nils D. Forkert[1]

[1] Department of Radiology and Hotchkiss Brains Institute,
University of Calgary, Calgary, AB, Canada
{phellan.renzo,nils.forkert}@ucalgary.ca
[2] Laboratory of Image Data Science, Institute of Computing,
University of Campinas, Campinas, SP, Brazil
peixinho@lids.ic.unicamp.br, afalcao@ic.unicamp.br

Abstract. Cerebrovascular diseases are one of the main causes of death and disability in the world. Within this context, fast and accurate automatic cerebrovascular segmentation is important for clinicians and researchers to analyze the vessels of the brain, determine criteria of normality, and identify and study cerebrovascular diseases. Nevertheless, automatic segmentation is challenging due to the complex shape, inhomogeneous intensity, and inter-person variability of normal and malformed vessels. In this paper, a deep convolutional neural network (CNN) architecture is used to automatically segment the vessels of the brain in time-of-flight magnetic resonance angiography (TOF MRA) images of healthy subjects. Bi-dimensional manually annotated image patches are extracted in the axial, coronal, and sagittal directions and used as input for training the CNN. For segmentation, each voxel is individually analyzed using the trained CNN by considering the intensity values of neighboring voxels that belong to its patch. Experiments were performed with TOF MRA images of five healthy subjects, using varying numbers of images to train the CNN. Cross validations revealed that the proposed framework is able to segment the vessels with an average Dice coefficient ranging from 0.764 to 0.786 depending on the number of images used for training. In conclusion, the results of this work suggest that CNNs can be used to segment cerebrovascular structures with an accuracy similar to other high-level segmentation methods.

Keywords: Vessel segmentation · Deep learning · Cerebrovascular segmentation · Convolutional neural networks

1 Introduction

Vascular diseases have led the ranking of major causes of death in the last fifteen years, according to reports of the world health organization (WHO) [1]. In particular, cerebrovascular diseases that lead to stroke were responsible for more

© Springer International Publishing AG 2017
M.J. Cardoso et al. (Eds.): CVII-STENT/LABELS 2017, LNCS 10552, pp. 39–46, 2017.
DOI: 10.1007/978-3-319-67534-3_5

than six million deaths only in 2015 [1]. Consequently, clinicians and researchers require fast and accurate tools, which aid them to detect, analyze, and treat cerebrovascular diseases, such as aneurysms, arteriovenous malformations (AVMs), and stenoses.

Segmentation of the vascular system in medical images allows clinicians to identify and isolate vessels from other surrounding types of tissue, thus, allowing better visualization and quantitative analysis. However, manual vessel segmentation is a time-consuming, error-prone task, which is subject to inter-observer variability. Consequently, research has been focused on developing faster and more accurate automatic vessel segmentation methods.

Lesage et al. [2] review paper lists a considerable number of automatic vessel segmentation approaches. The referenced methods range from approaches that are based on computing Hessian-based features of vessels, proposed by Frangi et al. [3] and Sato et al. [4], to atlas or model-based approaches, other feature-based methods, and extraction schemes, such as level-sets [5]. In all cases, different handcrafted features are used to guide the segmentation process, such as image intensities, Hessian eigenvalues, curvature values, gradient flow, and many others. It is the researcher who decides, based on experiments related to each particular application, which features are used to extract the to the most accurate segmentation results.

Deep convolutional neural networks (CNN) is a recent and popular strategy, with successful results solving different medical image analysis problems [6], which proposes to let the computer learn in an automatic and supervised manner, and decide which features are relevant to generate accurate segmentation results. Automatic vessel segmentation methods that use deep CNN have been used to segment 2D images of the retina [7], ultrasound images of the femoral region of the body [8], and computed tomography (CT) volumes of the liver [9], with a high performance in all cases.

To our knowledge, no study has been performed yet to adapt and apply deep CNN to segment the vessels of the brain, mainly due to the technical difficulties to obtain manually segmented brain datasets, the novelty of deep learning methods, and its associated long execution times. However, given the successful performance of CNN, as it has permeated the entire field of medical image analysis [6], this paper presents an initial strategy to apply deep CNN to segment the vascular system in time-of-flight magnetic resonance angiography (TOF MRA) images of the brain.

2   Vascular Segmentation of TOF MRA Images Using Deep CNN

TOF MRA is a medical imaging modality, which allows the acquisition of non-contrast enhanced images of the brain vascular system with a high spatial resolution [10]. TOF MRA images are affected by noise artifacts that do not allow the establishment of fixed intensity values to identify different types of tissue. Additionally, the intricate shape of the vascular tree, and its high inter-person variability, make it hard to define a common atlas that can be used for segmentation, as often conducted for different organs [11].

Given the variability of the intensity profile and complex shape of the vascular system in TOF MRA and other imaging modalities, defining suitable characteristics to identify and segment vessels represents a challenging problem. In order to solve this problem, deep CNN approaches have been used to let the computer discover and learn those characteristics by itself, in a supervised manner [8,12].

Traditionally, three-dimensional patches are extracted from a set of training images and used to optimize a deep CNN, which is then used to segment the vascular system, but they have not been tested for the purpose of segmenting cerebrovascular structures from 3D TOF MRA datasets yet.

2.1 CNN Architecture

Complex deep CNN architectures can lead to a possible over-fitting in the model learning, as well as significantly increasing the processing time, when considering TOF MRA images. For this reason, we propose a CNN architecture composed of only two convolutional layers (C1 and C2) and two fully connected layers (FC3 and FC4). This architecture is shown in Fig. 1.

The first convolutional layer, C1, contains 32 filters with 5×5 voxels receptive field, in a 2 voxels stride sliding (S1), sub sampled in a 3×3 voxels max-pooling (P1), in order to reduce translation variance. The next convolutional layer, C2, has a receptive field of 3×3 voxels, with 64 filters, and no sub sampling. In order to reduce the impact of the backpropagation vanishing problem, both convolutional layers are followed by a rectified linear activation (Relu).

After the convolutional layers, two more fully connected layers are added. The first fully connected layer, FC3, reduces the dimensionality from 256 ($2 \times 2 \times 64$) to 100 neurons, and FC4 can be seen as a decision layer that determines the likelihood of belonging to a vessel or not. These layers have hyperbolic tangent (Tanh) and sigmoid (Sigm) activation functions, respectively.

2.2 CNN Training

In order to identify the best weights for our model, we selected a balanced number of patches from vessel and non-vessel regions in our training dataset. In particular, we used a number of vessel and non-vessel patches equal to half the number of voxels in the vessel region of each dataset, in the axial, coronal, and sagittal planes. Through a mini-batch gradient descent approach, the squared error over the entire training set was minimized, considering a mini-batch of 50 elements. This learning approach is applied through 40 epochs, while considering a learning rate of 0.001 and a gradient momentum of 0.9.

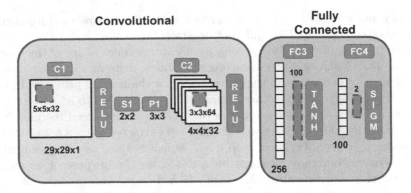

Fig. 1. Network architecture, composed of two convolutional layers, C1 and C2, and two fully connected layers, FC1 and FC2. After C1, we include a stride S1 of two voxels. All layers are also followed by a Relu, Tanh or Sigmoid function as indicated.

3   Materials and Methods

3.1   Data Acquisition and Image Preprocessing

Five TOF MRA datasets of healthy subjects were used to analyze and evaluate the proposed deep learning cerebrovascular segmentation method. The datasets were acquired on a 3T Intera MRI scanner (Philips, Eindhoven, the Netherlands) without application of contrast agent using a TE = 2.68 ms, a TR = 15.72 ms, a 20o flip angle, and a spatial resolution of $0.35 \times 0.35 \times 0.65\,\mathrm{mm}^3$. The datasets size is $512 \times 512 \times 120$ voxels.

For preprocessing, slab boundary artefact correction was performed using the method described by Kholmovski et al. [13] followed by intensity non-uniformity correction using the N3 algorithm [14]. A skull stripping algorithm [15] was also applied to mask the brain images and their corresponding binary segmentations. The vessels were manually segmented in each dataset by a medical expert based on the preprocessed TOF MRA datasets.

3.2   Classification

For all voxels inside the brain region, we define a cubic region of $29 \times 29 \times 29$ around this voxel, where the axial, coronal, and sagittal patches are extracted, as in [9]. All patches have $29 \times 29 \times 1$ voxels, as they are a bi-dimensional slice of each axis. Each patch is fed to the CNN, which calculates the vessel likelihood, so that three probability maps (for each orientation) are available after application of the CNN. A voxel is defined as a vessel voxel if at least one of the probability values (for the three directions) is above a threshold t and defined background otherwise. In this work, an empirically defined threshold of $t = 0.95$ was used for all experiments.

3.3   CNN Evaluation

The performance of the deep CNN is evaluated by selecting random sets of TOF MRA images for training. The number of images used for training is increased from one to four images, to evaluate if increasing the number of training images generates more accurate results. Initially, one TOF MRA image is randomly selected to train the CNN, which is used to segment the test image. The selected training image is different for each test image. Then, the number of training images is consecutively incremented up to four, always guaranteeing that the training set does not contain the test image.

The Dice similarity coefficient (DSC) [16] is used to compare the CNN-based segmentation and ground-truth manual segmentations, as it has been used in other cerebrovascular segmentation methods, thus, allowing an easier comparison. It is defined as $DSC = 2|A \cap B|/(|A| + |B|)$, where A and B represent the ground-truth and CNN segmentations, respectively.

A standard one-way analysis of variance (ANOVA) is applied to determine if the segmentation accuracies using an increasing number of images are statistically different, followed by the Tukey's honest significant difference procedure. The Statistical Package for the Social Sciences version 16.0 (SPSS Inc., Chicago, IL, USA) was used for this statistical analysis, and the criterion of statistical significance was set at $p < 0.05$.

3.4   Hardware Settings

Our deep CNN is implemented using version 2.7 of the python language, and the Theano 0.9.0 library [17]. Experiments are executed on a desktop computer with eight Intel(R) Core(TM) i7-4790 CPU @ 3.60 GHz processors, 32 GB of RAM memory, and graphic card GeForce GTX 745 (NVIDIA corp., United States), with 4 GB RAM memory. Testing and training were done using the graphic card and cuDNN extensions for faster processing [18].

4   Results

The results of the CNN approach for segmentation of vessels in TOF MRA images are reported in Table 1. The values correspond to the DSC when comparing the CNN segmentation with the manual ground-truths available for evaluation. Each row corresponds to a different dataset, and each column to the corresponding DSC when using the indicated number of images to train the deep neural network. The numbers in parenthesis identify the datasets used for training. Average DSC values, training and testing times are reported in the final rows.

The average DSC values for our deep learning approach vary between 0.764 and 0.786, depending on the number of images used for training. According to the ANOVA analysis, there is not enough evidence to guarantee that the resulting DSC values are significantly different (p >= 0.05). As expected, training times increase with the number of images used. The testing times are independent of the number of training images.

Table 1. DSC values for each dataset, when using a different number of images to train the deep neural network.

Dataset	1 image	2 images	3 images	4 images
1	0.774 (2)	0.763 (4, 5)	0.770 (2, 3, 4)	0.767
2	0.758 (5)	0.780 (3, 5)	0.759 (1, 3, 4)	0.765
3	0.769 (4)	0.784 (1, 4)	0.730 (1, 2, 4)	0.771
4	0.770 (2)	0.795 (1, 2)	0.804 (1, 3, 5)	0.781
5	0.751 (1)	0.809 (1, 3)	0.742 (1, 2, 4)	0.788
Average	**0.764±0.010**	**0.786±0.017**	**0.761±0.028**	**0.774±0.010**
Train (min)	40	65	92	120
Test (min)	30	30	30	30

5 Discussion

This paper presents a feasibility analysis of a deep CNN vessel segmentation method for TOF MRA images of the brain, with promising accuracy results. The CNN analyzes only in-plane neighboring voxels in the axial, coronal, and sagittal planes, and not full three-dimensional patches. Additionally, the Theano library with cuDNN extensions, and graphic card were used in the CNN implementation.

According to the executed statistical tests, using more images for training did not lead to a significant increase in segmentation accuracy. This result clearly highlights the benefit that a simple CNN, as described here, only needs very few well segmented ground truth datasets to achieve proper results, making an application in research or clinical settings more feasible.

Figure 2 shows 3D visualizations of the segmentation results for dataset 1, using the indicated number of images to train the proposed deep CNN. Visually, no considerable difference can be depicted between the segmentation results, confirming by the quantitative analysis. In general, it can be noted that large vessels are correctly identified. On the other hand, small vessels are partially affected by noise, such that their shape is not correctly delineated.

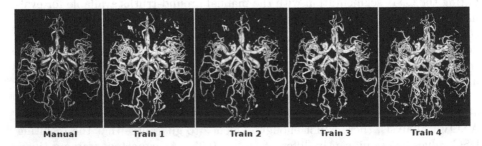

| Manual | Train 1 | Train 2 | Train 3 | Train 4 |

Fig. 2. 3D renderings of segmentation results for dataset 1 using a deep CNN trained with the indicated number of images.

As a limitation, it has to be noted that a small sample size with five TOF MRA images may not be enough to support general conclusions about the most suitable deep CNN architecture for vessel segmentation. However, the promising results of this initial analysis (as seen in Fig. 2) motivates further developments and analyses of this approach.

6 Conclusion

This paper presents a first feasibility analysis to apply deep CNN for automatic segmentation of the cerebrovascular system. Processing times were optimized by using bi-dimensional patches to identify vessels, and by taking advantage of the Theano library with cuDNN extensions, and graphic card of the system. No significant accuracy differences were found when using different numbers of images to train the deep CNN. The developed program calculates axial, coronal, and sagittal vessel probability maps and applies a fixed threshold to determine which voxels belong to vessels. It is expected that more complex approaches based on the calculated probability maps would lead to more accurate results.

Acknowledgement. This work was supported by Natural Sciences and Engineering Research Council of Canada (NSERC). Dr. Alexandre X. Falcão and MSc. Alan Peixinho thank CNPq 302970/2014-2 and FAPESP 2014/12236-1.

References

1. World Health Organization: The top 10 causes of death (2015)
2. Lesage, D., Angelini, E.D., Bloch, I., Funka-Lea, G.: A review of 3D vessel lumen segmentation techniques: models, features and extraction schemes. Med. Image Anal. **13**(6), 819–845 (2009)
3. Frangi, A.F., Niessen, W.J., Vincken, K.L., Viergever, M.A.: Multiscale vessel enhancement filtering. In: Wells, W.M., Colchester, A., Delp, S. (eds.) MICCAI 1998. LNCS, vol. 1496, pp. 130–137. Springer, Heidelberg (1998). doi:10.1007/BFb0056195
4. Sato, Y., Nakajima, S., Atsumi, H., Koller, T., Gerig, G., Yoshida, S., Kikinis, R.: 3D multi-scale line filter for segmentation and visualization of curvilinear structures in medical images. In: Troccaz, J., Grimson, E., Mösges, R. (eds.) CVRMed/MRCAS -1997. LNCS, vol. 1205, pp. 213–222. Springer, Heidelberg (1997). doi:10.1007/BFb0029240
5. Sethian, J.A.: Level Set Methods: Evolving Interfaces in Geometry, Fluid Mechanics, Computer Vision, and Materials Science. Cambridge University Press, Cambridge (1996)
6. Litjens, G., Kooi, T., Bejnordi, B.E., Setio, A.A.A., Ciompi, F., Ghafoorian, M., van der Laak, J.A., van Ginneken, B., Sánchez, C.I.: A survey on deep learning in medical image analysis. Med. Image Anal. **42**, 60–88 (2017)
7. Fu, H., Xu, Y., Wong, D.W.K., Liu, J.: Retinal vessel segmentation via deep learning network and fully-connected conditional random fields. In: IEEE 13th International Symposium on Biomedical Imaging, pp. 698–701. IEEE (2016)

8. Smistad, E., Løvstakken, L.: Vessel detection in ultrasound images using deep convolutional neural networks. In: Carneiro, G., Mateus, D., Peter, L., Bradley, A., Tavares, J.M.R.S., Belagiannis, V., Papa, J.P., Nascimento, J.C., Loog, M., Lu, Z., Cardoso, J.S., Cornebise, J. (eds.) LABELS/DLMIA -2016. LNCS, vol. 10008, pp. 30–38. Springer, Cham (2016). doi:10.1007/978-3-319-46976-8_4

9. Kitrungrotsakul, T., Han, X.H., Iwamoto, Y., Foruzan, A.H., Lin, L., Chen, Y.W.: Robust hepatic vessel segmentation using multi deep convolution network. In: SPIE Medical Imaging, International Society for Optics and Photonics, pp. 1013711–1013711 (2017)

10. Saloner, D.: The AAPM/RSNA physics tutorial for residents. an introduction to MR angiography. Radiographics 15(2), 453–465 (1995)

11. Forkert, N., Fiehler, J., Suniaga, S., Wersching, H., Knecht, S., Kemmling, A., et al.: A statistical cerebroarterial atlas derived from 700 MRA datasets. Methods Inf. Med. 52(6), 467–474 (2013)

12. Wu, A., Xu, Z., Gao, M., Buty, M., Mollura, D.J.: Deep vessel tracking: a generalized probabilistic approach via deep learning. In: IEEE 13th International Symposium on Biomedical Imaging, pp. 1363–1367. IEEE (2016)

13. Kholmovski, E.G., Alexander, A.L., Parker, D.L.: Correction of slab boundary artifact using histogram matching. J. Magn. Reson. Imaging 15(5), 610–617 (2002)

14. Sled, J.G., Zijdenbos, A.P., Evans, A.C.: A nonparametric method for automatic correction of intensity nonuniformity in MRI data. IEEE Trans. Med. Imaging 17(1), 87–97 (1998)

15. Forkert, N., Säring, D., Fiehler, J., Illies, T., Möller, D., Handels, H., et al.: Automatic brain segmentation in time-of-flight MRA images. Methods Inf. Med. 48(5), 399–407 (2009)

16. Dice, L.R.: Measures of the amount of ecologic association between species. Ecology 26(3), 297–302 (1945)

17. Bergstra, J., Breuleux, O., Bastien, F., Lamblin, P., Pascanu, R., Desjardins, G., Turian, J., Warde-Farley, D., Bengio, Y.: Theano: a CPU and GPU math compiler in Python. In: Proceedings of the 9th Python in Science Conference, pp. 1–7 (2010)

18. Chetlur, S., Woolley, C., Vandermersch, P., Cohen, J., Tran, J., Catanzaro, B., Shelhamer, E.: cuDNN: efficient primitives for deep learning. arXiv preprint arXiv:1410.0759 (2014)

VOIDD: Automatic Vessel-of-Intervention Dynamic Detection in PCI Procedures

Ketan Bacchuwar[1,2]($\boxtimes$), Jean Cousty[2], Régis Vaillant[1],
and Laurent Najman[2]

[1] General Electric Healthcare, Buc, France
ketan.bacchuwar@ge.com
[2] Université Paris-Est, LIGM, A3SI, ESIEE Paris, Noisy-le-Grand, France

Abstract. In this article, we present the work towards improving the overall workflow of the Percutaneous Coronary Interventions (PCI) procedures by capacitating the imaging instruments to precisely monitor the steps of the procedure. In the long term, such capabilities can be used to optimize the image acquisition to reduce the amount of dose or contrast media employed during the procedure. We present the automatic VOIDD algorithm to detect the vessel of intervention which is going to be treated during the procedure by combining information from the vessel image with contrast agent injection and images acquired during guidewire tip navigation. Due to the robust guidewire tip segmentation method, this algorithm is also able to automatically detect the sequence corresponding to guidewire navigation. We present an evaluation methodology which characterizes the correctness of the guide wire tip detection and correct identification of the vessel navigated during the procedure. On a dataset of 2213 images from 8 sequences of 4 patients, VOIDD identifies vessel-of-intervention with accuracy in the range of 88% or above and absence of tip with accuracy in range of 98% or above depending on the test case.

Keywords: Interventional cardiology · PCI procedure modeling · Image fusion · Coronary roadmap

1 Introduction

Percutaneous Coronary Intervention (PCI) is a procedure employed for the treatment of coronary artery stenosis. PCI is a very mature procedure relying on the deployment of a stent having the shape of the artery at the location of the stenosis. These procedures are performed under X-ray guidance with use of contrast agent. Consequently they also have side effects such as the injection of contrast agent based on iodine to the patient. The tolerance to this contrast agent is limited to some amount. The other side effect is the use of ionizing radiation which affects both the patient and the operator.

In the work presented here, we develop methods based on image processing to combine the information from fluoroscopic image sequences acquired at different steps of the procedure. More precisely, we consider two types of images: (i) the

© Springer International Publishing AG 2017
M.J. Cardoso et al. (Eds.): CVII-STENT/LABELS 2017, LNCS 10552, pp. 47–56, 2017.
DOI: 10.1007/978-3-319-67534-3_6

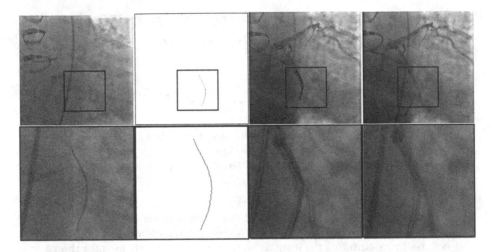

Fig. 1. VOIDD: (from left to right)Input image f; centerline of segmented guidewire tip; tip candidate (red) matched to vessel centerline (green) marked by pairings(blue); corresponding location (green) of guidewire tip(red) inside vessel. (Color figure online)

images from *reference sequence*, which are injected with contrast agent to depict the vasculature and (ii) the images from *navigation sequence*, which are acquired during the navigation of the tool and especially the guide wire, which is navigated from the ostia of the coronary artery down to the distal part after crossing the lesion. The imaging of the vessel with contrast agent provides information on the potential location of the stenosis. The ECG of the patient is recorded along with the images. Standard algorithm as [4] can then be used to identify the subset of the images where the coronary images are well opacified with the contrast agent. In this subset, a reference sequence of about 10 to 15 images is then selected that covers a full cardiac cycle and includes best opacified images. The navigation sequence is obtained with a low dose acquisition mode called fluoroscopy. The guidewire, a very thin (wire-like) object of diameter 0.014″ has two sections. The distal section, called as the tip, is more important and is enough radio opaque to be seen with low dose X-ray mode. Our aim is to automatically identify navigation sequence and determine the vessel-of-intervention which is going to be treated in the following steps of the PCI procedure, such as lesion reparation with angioplasty balloon, stenting, post-dilatation.

Several authors have worked on the task of segmenting the guidewire. For electrophysiology clinical application as in [7], the size of the tip of the catheters makes its contrast significant enough to enable the development of robust algorithms. For PCI application as in [5], the weak contrast of the guidewire body makes the task very challenging. Some manufacturers of interventional suite have proposed or are still including in their offer, applications which facilitate the visual appreciation of the relationship between the guidewire and the vessel. The main idea is to combine a suite of consecutive injected images which visualize the vessel along a cardiac cycle. These images are combined with the images obtained during tool navigation. The images between these different times are paired mostly based on the ECG and up to our knowledge neither the breathing motion, nor any slight deformation of the arteries caused by the introduction of the guidewire are compensated. In [8], the correspondence between a location identified in the fluoroscopic images acquired during tool navigation and the cine images which depict the injected vessels is searched. The addressed clinical need is the registration of intra-vascular images acquired with a sensor placed along the guidewire with the vessel. By this means, the operator can easily correlate the readings of the angiographic images and the intravascular images/signals. In this situation, a full application is developed with a specific acquisition workflow with the different steps of the image acquisition and processing being done based on landmark points and appropriate images selected by an operator.

The main contribution of this article is the proposition and the assessment of a method, called VOIDD, to automatically detect the so-called vessel-of-intervention during the navigation of the guidewire. More precisely this algorithm is able to recognize from the stream of fluoroscopic images following the acquisition of the reference sequence, the period corresponding to the guidewire navigation and to exploit it to determine the vessel-of-intervention (see Fig. 1). In order to reach this goal a general tracking algorithm is proposed and explained in Sect. 2.1. This algorithm relies on features extracted from the navigation and reference images. Various methods can be adopted or designed to extract these features to be used with our general tracking algorithm. In this article, these features consists of vessel tree segmentation and of guidewire tip location candidates detection with advanced approaches involving the use of min tree [9]. Graph-based matching approaches derived from [2] are used to match the guidewire tip with the vessel. These developments have been evaluated on 4 patient dataset. We present an evaluation methodology which characterizes the correctness of the guide wire tip detection and the correct identification of the vessel navigated during the procedures. On a dataset of 4 patients, VOIDD identifies vessel-of-intervention with accuracy in the range of 88% or above and absence of tip with accuracy in range of 98% or above depending on the test case.

2   Vessel-of-Intervention Dynamic Detection (VOIDD) Algorithm

In this section, we first elaborate the general tracking framework of the VOIDD algorithm proposed in this article (in Sect. 2.1). We then explain (in Sect. 2.2) how to extract the features (from the *reference sequence* and the *navigation sequence*), which are used by the VOIDD algorithm.

2.1   General Tracking Framework

We aim to obtain the vessel-of-intervention by making a smart correspondence between the input guidewire navigation sequence and the reference sequence. Therefore, we propose an algorithm, called VOIDD, that is able to simultaneously detect the guidewire tip in the navigation sequence and the section of the

---

Algorithm 1. VOIDD

Data: Guidewire navigation sequence and reference sequence $\mathcal{R}$
Result: T_{vessel} Track of vessel-of-intervention and detected guidewire tips

1 Initialize $\mathcal{T}, T_{best} = \emptyset$ and d_{best} to track assignment distance threshold ;
2 **foreach** *image I in the guidewire navigation sequence* **do**
3     $\mathcal{P} := \textbf{ExtractFeaturePairs}(I, \mathcal{R})$;
    // feature pairs are ranked in decreasing order of matching score
4   **foreach** $P \in \mathcal{P}$ **do**
5   **foreach** $T \in \mathcal{T}$ **do**
6           $d_{ij} := T \to \textbf{TrackAssignmentDistance}(P)$;
7   **if** $d_{ij} < d_{best}$ **then**
8              $T_{best} := T$; $d_{best} := d_{ij}$;
9   **if** $T_{best} \neq \emptyset$ **then**
10   **AssignTrack**(T_{best}, P);
11   **if** *(P $\to$ TrackNotAssigned())* **then**
12          $T_{new} := \textbf{MakeTrack}(P)$; $\mathcal{T} \to$ AddTrack(T_{new}) ;
13   Reset(T_{best}, d_{best});
14 $T_{vessel} = \mathcal{T} \to$ LongestTrack() ;

---

coronary artery tree in which the guidewire is currently navigating in the reference sequence. From a broader perspective, the algorithm consists of: (i) detecting feature pairs from the navigation and reference sequence; (ii) grouping these feature pairs into tracks, a track being a sequence of features that are spatially consistent in time; (iii) selecting the most relevant track as the detected vessel-of-intervention. A feature pair is made of two corresponding curves. The first one, called a *tip candidate*, is extracted from the guidewire navigation sequence and possibly corresponds to the guidewire tip in the fluoroscopic image. The second one, called a vessel-of-intervention *(VOI) candidate* is obtained from the reference sequence and is a part of the coronary vessels that optimally fits the associated tip candidate. The precise description of the VOIDD algorithm and of the feature pairs extraction is given in Algorithm 1 and in the Sect. 2.2 respectively.

VOIDD algorithm manages a dictionary of tracks $\mathcal{T}$, where each track $T \in \mathcal{T}$ is a sequence of feature pairs, with at most one pair per image in the guidewire navigation sequence. For each time step of the navigation sequence, the essence of the algorithm lies in optimally assigning the best detected feature pair to the existing tracks. To this end, the feature pairs are ranked in decreasing order of matching score, provided by the feature extraction algorithm. Then, a distance between feature pair and track, called the *track assignment distance* (TAD) (described in the Sect. 2.3), is considered to optimally assign the considered feature pair to the track which is at least distance. A TAD threshold is computed as the theoretically maximum possible value of TAD based on the length of the guidewire tip and maximum observed guidewire speed. If TAD to the closest track is above the TAD threshold then the feature pair is not assigned to any existing track but is used to initialize a new track in $\mathcal{T}$. Once all the frames in the navigation sequence are processed, the longest track (*i.e.* track with maximum feature pairs) is selected as the vessel-of-intervention.

2.2 Feature Pairs Extraction

This section elaborates the extraction of the feature pairs, which are associations between the images of the navigation sequence and the images of the reference sequence. First, we explain the *tip candidate* extraction by segmentation and morphological thinning. This is followed by the extraction of centerline of the injected vessels to obtain vessel graph. Finally, we present the matching part to find the possible associations (the *VOI candidates*) of the tip candidate in the vessel graph. However, different methods can be adopted or designed to obtain these feature pairs.

Tip candidate extraction. Guidewire tip appears as contrasted thin and elongated object in the fluoroscopic image. We are interested to segment the guidewire tip, using a component tree called min tree. The min tree [9] structures all the connected components of the lower-level sets of the grayscale image based on inclusion relationship. We assign to any connected component C of the min tree $\mathcal{M}$, a shape attribute characterizing the shape and structural properties of guidewire tip. Then, the considered attribute $\mathcal{A}$ describes the elongation of the components. For any component C, $\mathcal{A}(C) = (\pi \times l_{max}(C)^2)/|C|$, where $|.|$ represents cardinality and $l_{max}(C)$ is the length of the largest axis of the best fitting ellipse for the connected component C. Since the guidewire tip is thin and long, the component corresponding to the tip have high value of attribute $\mathcal{A}$. A mere thresholding of the elongation $\mathcal{A}$ is not sufficient, often giving other long and elongated (unwanted) objects like pacing lead and filled catheters. Indeed, these objects have higher elongation value than the guidewire tip. Hence, according to physical properties of the guidewire tip, we set a upper bound value t_{max} on $\mathcal{A}$ to maximum possible elongation value of the guidewire tip, to ensure that extracted components contain guidewire tip. Even with this upperbound threshold keeping the most elongated component does not always lead to the desired tip. Based on min tree structure, the nested connected components that satisfy the criterion are filtered to preserve the component with largest area (taking aid of the inclusion relationship). Therefore, we adopt the shaping framework [10] that allows us to efficiently extract significant connected components. The extracted components constitute the tip candidates. Shaping extensively uses the min tree structure to regularize the attributes and to select the relevant components. In order to facilitate matching, we perform skeletonization [3] of the selected connected component(s) to obtain centerline of the tip candidates. Figure 1 shows the obtained centerline of segmented guidewire tip from the input image. This centerline of the tip candidate $\mathcal{C}$ is modeled as a discrete polygonal curve.

Vessel centerline extraction. The coronary vessels from each fluoroscopic image in the reference sequence are enhanced using a Hessian based technique [6] followed by centerline extraction using Non-Maximum Supression and hysteresis thresholding. We represent these centerlines of vessels by a non-directed graph $\mathcal{X}$ where the nodes are represented by bifurcations whereas the edges refer to curvilinear centerlines. Apparent bifurcations resulting from superimposing vessels in 2D X-ray projections also form nodes. Such graph is computed for each frame in the reference sequence providing us with a representation for each phase of the cardiac cycle.

Matching. An important step in the task of vessel-of-intervention detection is to designate possible desirable associations of the corresponding location of the guidewire tip inside the injected vessel. We refer to these locations in vessels as *vessel-of-interest* (VOI) candidates. This step refers to building the correspondences between the centerline of each tip candidate $\mathcal{C}$ extracted from navigation sequence and the corresponding centerlines of the vessels $\mathcal{X}$ extracted from reference sequence by taking into account ECG information. We adopt the curve pairing algorithm of [2] to perform this task. It is required to define a curve-to-curve distance to compare the two sets of curves mentioned above. We use a discrete version of Fréchet distance [1] as it takes into account the topological structures of the curves. Thus, this Fréchet distance is computed from a mapping between two ordered sets of discrete polygonal curves denoted by $\mathcal{C}$ and by X_C, respectively. Imposed non-decreasing surjective mappings (reparameterization mapping) in computation of Fréchet distance takes into account the order of points along curves. This order also helps us in curve pairing described below, to give scan direction along the curves.

The above step requires the selection of every admissible curve X_C in graph $\mathcal{X}$. A curve in $\mathcal{X}$ is a path between two nodes, without visiting the same edge twice. In order to restrict computational complexity of search, we restrict the set of admissible curves to be in the neighborhood of the tip candidate extremities $\mathcal{C}[1]$ and $\mathcal{C}[n]$ and we construct all possible paths between them in the graph. Indeed, these admissible curves are the VOI candidates. These VOI candidates, together with the tip candidate $\mathcal{C}$, is a *set of feature pairs* $\mathcal{P} = \{(\mathcal{C}, X_C) \mid X_C \text{ is some curve in } \mathcal{X} \text{ matched to } \mathcal{C}\}$, which are further filtered and ranked according to the shape similarity measure to prefer VOI candidates with higher shape resemblance to the tip candidate. This term is computed from residual Fréchet distance after the 2D transformation [2]. The set of feature pairs $\mathcal{P}$ is computed for each image in the guidewire tip navigation sequence by performing the matching with the vessel graph of the corresponding cardiac phase.

2.3   Track Assignment Distance (TAD)

The TAD is computed as a distance between a proposed feature pair $P = (\mathcal{C}, X_C)$ and a track T. It is the average of tip candidate distance, VOI candidate distance and graph distance. The tip candidate distance and the VOI candidate distance are computed between the proposed feature pair and the latest added feature pair of T. The tip candidate distance accounts for the geometrical shift between the two tip candidates. The VOI candidate distance measures the mean Euclidean distance between the end-points of the VOI candidates. The graph distance is computed between the proposed feature pair and the latest iso cardiac phase feature pair in T. It is the length of the path between two VOI candidates from two images in the same cardiac phase obtained from different cardiac cycles. The VOI candidate distance and the graph distance helps to preserve temporal coherency in the tracks. We transform these three distances with exponential functions so that they belong in the same range $[0–1[$. The parameters of these exponential functions are set according to the length of the guidewire tip.

3   Results

This section reports the performance of the VOIDD algorithm to detect the vessel-of-intervention and assesses its potential to identify the guidewire tip navigation sequence. An expert user annotated (with cross-validation) the center-line of the branch of the artery navigated by the guidewire tip as the ground truth. Ground truth was marked by a single expert user using a semi-automatic software guided by the vessel centerline extracted by the method in Sect. 2.2. This ground truth centerline is modeled as a discrete polygonal curve $GT = [GT[1] \cdots GT[M]]$. A VOI candidate X selected by VOIDD is similarly modeled as $X = [X[1] \cdots X[N]]$ with N equidistantly spaced points chosen at sub-pixel resolution. To assess the correctness of the automatically detected vessel, we consider the following target-to-registration (TRE) error between X and GT given by, $TRE = \frac{1}{N}\sum_{i=1}^{i=N} \min_{\forall j \in 1 \cdots M-1} |d(X_C[i], GT(j, j+1))|$, where $GT(j, j+1)$ refers to the segment between point $GT[j]$ and $GT[j+1]$ and d refers to point to segment distance converted to mm using known detector pixel size. If the tip is correctly paired to vessel-of-intervention then this TRE error is governed by the usual small difference between the estimated centerline and the expert marked vessel centerline. The algorithm chosen tip and vessel-of-intervention are considered as a *correct detection* if the corresponding TRE error is less than 0.5 mm. If TRE error is more than 0.5 mm, we consider that we have a *wrong detection*. If the input image contains guidewire tip, but the algorithm do not provide any detection, then the TRE error cannot be computed and a *missed detection* is reported. This may occur due to the fact that, sometimes the tip appears to be very blurred due to its sudden movement or due to reduced visibility of the tip caused by small contrast media injection to guide the navigation. In order to further evaluate the efficacy of the algorithm to identify the navigation sequence, we analyze its robustness to detect navigated vessel in sequence with no guidewire tip. In such sequence, if the algorithm detects a vessel-of-intervention in an image, it is counted as a *false detection*.

Sequences A1, B1, C1 and D1 in Table 1 show the efficacy of VOIDD algorithm to detect vessel-of-intervention during guidewire navigation in 4 patients and over 1513 images. In summary, VOIDD algorithm is able to correctly determine the location of tip in the vessel-of-intervention with an accuracy of around 88%–92%. The sequences A2, B2, C2 and D2 in the Table 1 portray the efficiency to identify navigation sequence over 690 images when guidewire tip is

Table 1. Performance of VOIDD algorithm on 4 patients

Patient	Sequence	Number of frames	Frames with tips	Correct detection	Wrong detection	Missed detection	False Detection
A	A1	164	164	92.07%	0%	7.92%	NA
B	B1	706	706	88.52%	5.80%	5.66%	NA
C	C1	449	449	92.20%	5.12%	2.67%	NA
D	D1	204	204	89.70%	2.94%	7.35%	NA
A	A2	156	0	NA	NA	NA	1.28%
B	B2	172	0	NA	NA	NA	0.58%
C	C2	264	0	NA	NA	NA	1.50%
D	D2	98	0	NA	NA	NA	2.04%

absent in the fluoroscopic images. The VOIDD algorithm is able to detect these sequences as sequence without guidewire tip with accuracy of 98%–99%. Analyzing the navigation sequence detection accuracy of VOIDD, we can use it to automatically detect the arrival of the guidewire tip. The parameters involved in various stages of the algorithm *e.g.* tip candidate extraction or TAD were designed based on the physical properties of guidewire tip, permissible speed of advancement of guidewire. Current implementation runs in average 0.33 s for tracking on a Intel Core i7 cadenced at 2.80 GHz. Videos are available as supplementary material[1]. Figure 2 shows the vessel of intervention obtained by the VOIDD algorithm and corresponding ground truth on left.

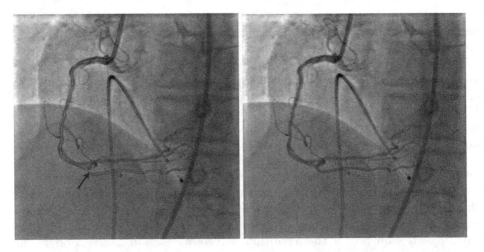

Fig. 2. VOIDD result: ground truth (in green) and vessel of intervention obtained from longest track (in red). In ground truth, the catheter is marked by the expert but not part of the tracked vessel because the guidewire tip is not detected when it is still inside the catheter. In this case, the vessel makes a very tight loop (blue arrow) in the bottom. In the tracking, we fail to detect this loop. (Color figure online)

---

[1] https://voidd-miccai17.github.io/.

4   Conclusion and Future Work

We proposed in this paper a framework to determine the vessel-of-intervention in fluoroscopic images during the PCI procedures. We also demonstrate the segmentation of the guidewire tip and the accuracy of its detection. This algorithm has the potential to be part of the software embarked by X-ray imaging systems and capable of automatically monitoring the successive steps of the procedure in view of continuously adapting the system behavior to the user needs. For instance, the guidewire tip tracking can be used to determine the phases related to the navigation of the guidewire, adding more semantic information, hence can be a first step towards smart semantic monitoring of the procedure. In order to perform such semantic analysis of the procedure, it is important to know the position of different interventional tools like guidewire tip, marker balls, balloon and this application opens the doors to ease the segmentation of these objects in the vessel-of-intervention. Encouraging results have been obtained with success rate above 88% for vessel of intervention detection. Future work includes the collection of additional clinical cases. In the longer term, we will investigate the detection of the other major tools and their integration into a semantic model of the procedure.

References

1. Alt, H., Godau, M.: Measuring the resemblance of polygonal curves. In: Eighth Annual Symposium on Computational Geometry, pp. 102–109. ACM (1992)
2. Benseghir, T., Malandain, G., Vaillant, R.: A tree-topology preserving pairing for 3D/2D registration. IJCARS **10**(6), 913–923 (2015)
3. Couprie, M., Bertrand, G.: Discrete topological transformations for image processing. In: Brimkov, V.E., Barneva, R.P. (eds.) Digital Geometry Algorithms. LNCVB, vol. 2, pp. 73–107. Springer, Dordrecht (2012). doi:10.1007/978-94-007-4174-4_3
4. Hoffmann, M., Müller, S., Kurzidim, K., Strobel, N., Hornegger, J.: Robust identification of contrasted frames in fluoroscopic images. In: Handels, H., Deserno, T.M., Meinzer, H.-P., Tolxdorff, T. (eds.) Bildverarbeitung für die Medizin 2015. I, pp. 23–28. Springer, Heidelberg (2015). doi:10.1007/978-3-662-46224-9_6
5. Honnorat, N., Vaillant, R., Paragios, N.: Graph-based guide-wire segmentation through fusion of contrast-enhanced and fluoroscopic images. In: ISBI 2012, pp. 948–951. IEEE (2012)
6. Krissian, K., Malandain, G., Ayache, N., Vaillant, R., Trousset, Y.: Model-based detection of tubular structures in 3D images. CVIU **80**(2), 130–171 (2000)
7. Milletari, F., Belagiannis, V., Navab, N., Fallavollita, P.: Fully automatic catheter localization in C-arm images using $\ell 1$-sparse coding. In: Golland, P., Hata, N., Barillot, C., Hornegger, J., Howe, R. (eds.) MICCAI 2014. LNCS, vol. 8674, pp. 570–577. Springer, Cham (2014). doi:10.1007/978-3-319-10470-6_71
8. Prasad, M., Cassar, A., Fetterly, K.A., Bell, M., Theessen, H., Ecabert, O., Bresnahan, J.F., Lerman, A.: Co-registration of angiography and intravascular ultrasound images through image-based device tracking. Cathet. Cardiovasc. Interv. **88**(7), 1077–1082 (2015)

9. Salembier, P., Wilkinson, M.H.: Connected operators. IEEE Signal Process. Mag. **26**(6), 136–157 (2009)
10. Xu, Y., Géraud, T., Najman, L.: Morphological filtering in shape spaces: applications using tree-based image representations. In: ICPR, pp. 485–488. IEEE (2012)

Second International Workshop on Large-Scale Annotation of Biomedical Data and Expert Label Synthesis, LABELS 2017

Exploring the Similarity of Medical Imaging Classification Problems

Veronika Cheplygina[1,2(✉)], Pim Moeskops[1], Mitko Veta[1],
Behdad Dashtbozorg[1], and Josien P.W. Pluim[1,3]

[1] Medical Image Analysis, Department of Biomedical Engineering,
Eindhoven University of Technology, Eindhoven, The Netherlands
v.cheplygina@tue.nl
[2] Biomedical Imaging Group Rotterdam,
Departments of Radiology and Medical Informatics,
Erasmus Medical Center, Rotterdam, The Netherlands
[3] Image Sciences Institute, University Medical Center Utrecht,
Utrecht, The Netherlands

Abstract. Supervised learning is ubiquitous in medical image analysis. In this paper we consider the problem of meta-learning – predicting which methods will perform well in an unseen classification problem, given previous experience with other classification problems. We investigate the first step of such an approach: how to quantify the similarity of different classification problems. We characterize datasets sampled from six classification problems by performance ranks of simple classifiers, and define the similarity by the inverse of Euclidean distance in this meta-feature space. We visualize the similarities in a 2D space, where meaningful clusters start to emerge, and show that the proposed representation can be used to classify datasets according to their origin with 89.3% accuracy. These findings, together with the observations of recent trends in machine learning, suggest that meta-learning could be a valuable tool for the medical imaging community.

1 Introduction

Imagine that you are a researcher in medical image analysis, and you have experience with machine learning methods in applications A, B, and C. Now imagine that a colleague, who just started working on application D, asks your advice on what type of methods to use, since trying all of them is too time-consuming. You will probably ask questions like "How much data do you have?" to figure out what advice to give. In other words, your perception of the similarity of problem D with problems A, B and C, is going to influence what kind of "rules of thumb" you will tell your colleague to use.

In machine learning, this type of process is called *meta-learning*, or "learning to learn". In this meta-learning problem, the samples are the different datasets A, B and C, and the labels are the best-performing methods on each dataset. Given this data, we want to know what the best-performing method for D will be.

© Springer International Publishing AG 2017
M.J. Cardoso et al. (Eds.): CVII-STENT/LABELS 2017, LNCS 10552, pp. 59–66, 2017.
DOI: 10.1007/978-3-319-67534-3_7

The first step is to characterize the datasets in a meta-feature space. The meta-features can be defined by properties of the datasets, such as sample size, or by performances of simple classifiers [1–3]. Once the meta-feature space is defined, dataset similarity can be defined to be inversely proportional to the Euclidean distances within this space, and D can be labeled, for example, by a nearest neighbor classifier.

Despite the potential usefulness of this approach, the popularity of meta-learning has decreased since its peak around 15 years ago. To the best of our knowledge, meta-learning is not widely known in the medical imaging community, although methods for predicting the quality of registration [4] or segmentation [5] can be considered to meta-learn within a single application. In part, meta-learning seems less relevant today because of the superior computational resources. However, with the advent of deep learning and the number of choices to be made in terms of architecture and other parameters, we believe that meta-learning is worth revisiting in the context of its use in applications in medical image analysis.

In this paper we take the first steps towards a meta-learning approach for classification problems in medical image analysis. More specifically, we investigate the construction of a meta-feature space, where datasets known to be similar (i.e. sampled from the same classification problem), form clusters. We represent 120 datasets sampled from six different classification problems by performances of six simple classifiers and propose several methods to embed the datasets into a two-dimensional space. Furthermore, we evaluate whether a classifier is able to predict which classification problem a dataset is sampled from, based on only a few normalized classifier performances. Our results show that even in this simple meta-feature space, clusters are beginning to emerge and 89.3% of the datasets can be classified correctly. We conclude with a discussion of the limitations of our approach, the steps needed for future research, and the potential value for the medical imaging community.

2   Methods

In what follows, we make the distinction between a "classification problem" - a particular database associated with extracted features, and a "dataset" - a subsampled version of this original classification problem.

We assume we are given datasets $\{(D_i, M_i)\}_1^n$, where D_i is a dataset from some supervised classification problem, and M_i is a meta-label that reflects some knowledge about D_i. For example, M_i could be the best-performing (but time-consuming) machine learning method for D_i. For this initial investigation, M_i is defined as the original classification problem D_i is sampled from.

We represent each dataset D_i by performances of k simple classifiers. Each of the n D_is is therefore represented by an k-dimensional vector $\mathbf{x}_i$ which together form a $n \times k$ meta-dataset A_k. Due to different inherent class overlap, the values in A_k might not be meaningful to compare to each other. To address this problem, we propose to transform the values of each $\mathbf{x}_i$ by:

- Normalizing the values to zero mean and unit variance, creating a meta-dataset N_k
- Ranking the values between 1 and k, creating a meta-dataset R_k. In cases of ties, we use average ranks.

The final step is to embed the meta-datasets A_k, N_k and R_k in a 2D space for visualization, to obtain A_2, N_2 and R_2. We use two types of embedding: multi-dimensional scaling (MDS) [6] and t-stochastic nearest neighbor embedding (t-SNE) [7]. These embeddings can help to understand complementary properties of the data. MDS emphasizes large distances, and is therefore good at pointing out outliers, whereas t-SNE emphasizes small distances, potentially creating more meaningful visualizations. An overview of the approach is shown in Fig. 1.

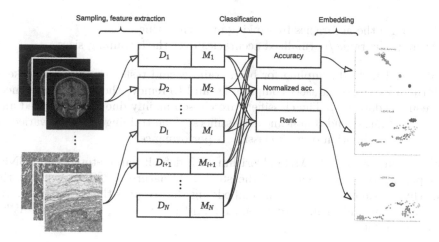

Fig. 1. Overview of the method.

3   Experiments

Data and Setup. We sample datasets from six classification problems, described in Table 1. The problems are segmentation or detection problems, the number of samples (pixels or voxels) is therefore much higher than the number of images. We sample each classification problem 20 times by selecting 70% of the subjects for training, and 30% of the subjects for testing, to generate $n = 120$ datasets for the embedding. For each of dataset, we do the following:

- Subsample {100, 300, 1K, 3K, 10K} pixels/voxels from the training subjects
- Train $k = 6$ classifiers on each training set: nearest mean, linear discriminant, quadratic discriminant, logistic regression, 1-nearest neighbor and decision tree
- Subsample 10 K pixels/voxels from the test subjects
- Evaluate accuracy on the test set, to obtain 5×6 accuracies

Table 1. Classification problems described by type of image, number of images (subjects), number of classes and number and type of features: "Classical" = intensity and texture-based, "CNN" = defined by output of the fully-connected layer of a convolutional neural network.

Dataset	Type	Images	Classes	Features
Tissue [8]	Brain MR	20	7	768, CNN [9]
Mitosis, MitosisNorm [10]	Histopathology	12	2	200, CNN [11]
Vessel [12]	Retinal	20	2	29, Classical [13]
ArteryVein [14]	Retinal	20	2	30, Classical [14]
Microaneurysm [15]	Retinal	381	2	30, Classical

- Transform the accuracies by ranking or normalizing
- Average the ranks/normalized accuracies over the 5 training sizes

We use balanced sampling for both training and test sets, in order to keep performances across datasets comparable (and to remove the "easy" differences between the datasets). The classifiers are chosen mainly due to their speed and diversity (3 linear and 3 non-linear classifiers). The training sizes are varied to get a better estimation of each classifier's performance.

Embedding. We use the MDS algorithm with default parameters[1], and t-SNE[2] with perplexity = 5. Because of the stochastic nature of t-SNE, we run the algorithm 10 times, and select the embedding that returns the lowest error. We apply each embedding method to A_k, N_k and R_k, creating embeddings A_2^{tsne}, A_2^{mds} and so forth.

Classification. To quantify the utility of each embedding, we also perform a classification experiment. We train a 1-nearest neighbor classifier to distinguish between the different classification problems, based on the meta-representation. The classifiers are trained with a random subset of {5, 10, 20, 40, 60} meta-samples 5 times, and accuracy is evaluated on the remaining meta-samples.

4 Results

Embedding. The embeddings are shown in Fig. 2. The embeddings based on accuracy are the best at discovering the true structure. Although we sampled the datasets in a balanced way in an attempt to remove some differences in accuracy, it is clear that some problems have larger or smaller class overlap, and therefore consistently lower or higher performances. Both t-SNE and MDS are able to recover this structure.

---

[1] http://prtools.org/.

[2] https://lvdmaaten.github.io/tsne/.

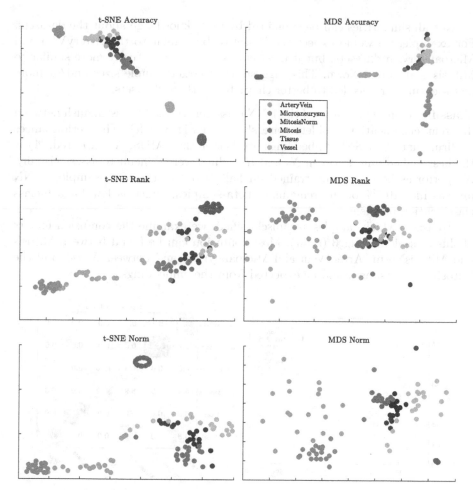

Fig. 2. 2D embeddings of the datasets with t-SNE (left) and MDS (right), based on accuracy (top), ranks (middle) and scaling (bottom).

Looking at N_2 and R_2, t-SNE appears to be slightly better at separating clusters of datasets from the same classification problem. This is particularly clear when looking at the ArteryVein datasets. Visually it is difficult to judge whether N_2 or R_2 provides a more meaningful embedding, which is why it is instructive to look at how a classifier would perform with each of the embeddings.

Looking at the different clusters, several patterns start to emerge. ArteryVein and Microaneurysm are quite similar to each other, likely to to the similarity of the images and the features used. Furthermore, Mitosis and MitosisNorm datasets are quite similar to each other, which is expected, because the same images but with different normalization are used. The Tissue dataset is often the most isolated from the others, being the only dataset based on 3D MR images.

Not all similarities can be explained by prior knowledge about the datasets. For example, we would expect the Vessel to be similar to the ArteryVein and Microaneurysm datasets, but it most embeddings it is actually more similar to Mitosis and MitosisNorm. This suggests that larger sample sizes and/or more meta-features are needed to better characterize these datasets.

Classification. The results of the 1-NN classifier, trained to distinguish between different classification problems, are shown in Fig. 3 (left). The performances confirm that the t-SNE embeddings are better than MDS. As expected, A_2 is the best embedding. Between N_2 and R_2, which were difficult to assess visually, N_2 performs better. When trained on half ($=60$) of the meta-samples, 1-NN misclassifies 10.7% of the remaining meta-samples, which is low for a 6-class classification problem.

To assess which samples are misclassified, we examine the confusion matrix of this classifier in Fig. 3 (right). Most confusion can be found between Mitosis and MitosisNorm, ArteryVein and Microaneyrism and between Vessel and the Mitosis datasets, as would be expected from the embeddings.

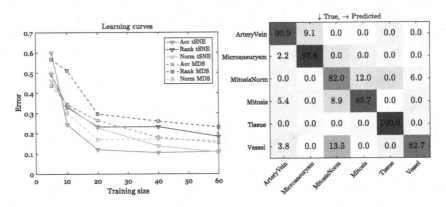

Fig. 3. Left: Learning curves of 1-NN classifiers trained on different-size samples from six meta-datasets. Right: confusion matrix of classifier trained on 60 samples from N_2^{tsne}. Each cell shows what % of the true class (row) is classified as (column).

5   Discussion and Conclusions

We presented an approach to quantify the similarity of medical imaging datasets, by representing each dataset by performances of six linear and non-linear classifiers. Even though we used small samples from each dataset and only six classifiers, this representation produced meaningful clusters and was reasonably successful (89.3% accuracy) in predicting the origin of each dataset. This demonstrates the potential of using this representation in a meta-learning approach, with the goal of predicting which machine learning method will be effective for a previously unseen dataset.

The main limitation is the use of artificial meta-labels, based on each dataset's original classification problem. Ideally the labels should reflect the best-performing method on the dataset. However, we would not expect the best-performing method to change for different samplings of the same dataset. Therefore, since we observe clusters with these artificial meta-labels, we also expect to observe clusters if more realistic meta-labels are used. Validating the approach with classifier-based meta-labels is the next step for a more practical application of this method.

Furthermore, we considered features as immutable properties of the classification problem. By considering the features as fixed, our approach would only be able to predict which classifier to apply to these already extracted features. However, due to recent advances in CNNs, where no explicit distinction is made between feature extraction and classification, we would want to start with the raw images. A challenge that needs to be addressed is how to represent the datasets at this point: for example, performances of classifiers on features extracted by CNNs pretrained on external data, or by some intrinsic, non-classifier-based characteristics. In a practical application, perceived similarity of the images (for example, obtained via crowdsourcing) could be used in addition to these features.

Despite these limitations, we believe this study reaches a more important goal: that of increasing awareness about meta-learning, which is largely overlooked by the medical imaging community. One opportunity is to use meta-learning jointly with transfer learning or domain adaptation, which have similar goals of transferring knowledge from a source dataset to a target dataset. For example, pretraining a CNN on the source, and extracting features on the target, is a form of transfer. In this context, meta-learning could be used to study which source datasets should be used for the transfer: for example, a single most similar source, or a selection of several, diverse sources.

Another opportunity is to learn more general rules of thumb for "what works when" by running the same feature extraction and classification pipelines on different medical imaging datasets, such as challenge datasets. In machine learning, this type of comparison is already being facilitated by OpenML [16], a large experiment database allows running different classification pipelines on already extracted features. We believe that a similar concept for medical imaging, that would also include preprocessing and feature extraction steps, would be a valuable resource for the community.

References

1. Vilalta, R., Drissi, Y.: A perspective view and survey of meta-learning. Artif. Intell. Rev. **18**, 77–95 (2002)
2. Duin, R.P.W., Pekalska, E., Tax, D.M.J.: The characterization of classification problems by classifier disagreements. Int. Conf. Pattern Recogn. **1**, 141–143 (2004)
3. Cheplygina, V., Tax, D.M.J.: Characterizing multiple instance datasets. In: Feragen, A., Pelillo, M., Loog, M. (eds.) SIMBAD 2015. LNCS, vol. 9370, pp. 15–27. Springer, Cham (2015). doi:10.1007/978-3-319-24261-3_2

4. Muenzing, S.E.A., van Ginneken, B., Viergever, M.A., Pluim, J.P.W.: DIRBoost-an algorithm for boosting deformable image registration: application to lung CT intra-subject registration. Med. Image Anal. **18**(3), 449–459 (2014)

5. Gurari, D., Jain, S.D., Betke, M., Grauman, K.: Pull the plug? predicting if computers or humans should segment images. In: Computer Vision and Pattern Recognition, pp. 382–391 (2016)

6. Cox, T.F., Cox, M.A.: Multidimensional Scaling. CRC Press, Boca Raton (2000)

7. van der Maaten, L., Hinton, G.: Visualizing data using t-SNE. J. Mach. Learn. Res. **9**, 2579–2605 (2008)

8. Landman, B.A., et al.: MICCAI 2012 Workshop on Multi-Atlas Labeling. CreateSpace Independent Publishing Platform (2012)

9. Moeskops, P., Viergever, M.A., Mendrik, A.M., de Vries, L.S., Benders, M.J., Išgum, I.: Automatic segmentation of MR brain images with a convolutional neural network. IEEE Trans. Med. Imaging **35**(5), 1252–1261 (2016)

10. Veta, M., Van Diest, P.J., Willems, S.M., Wang, H., Madabhushi, A., Cruz-Roa, A., Gonzalez, F., Larsen, A.B., Vestergaard, J.S., Dahl, A.B., et al.: Assessment of algorithms for mitosis detection in breast cancer histopathology images. Med. Image Anal. **20**(1), 237–248 (2015)

11. Veta, M., van Diest, P.J., Jiwa, M., Al-Janabi, S., Pluim, J.P.W.: Mitosis counting in breast cancer: object-level interobserver agreement and comparison to an automatic method. PLoS ONE **11**(8), e0161286 (2016)

12. Staal, J., Abràmoff, M.D., Niemeijer, M., Viergever, M.A., van Ginneken, B.: Ridge-based vessel segmentation in color images of the retina. IEEE Trans. Med. Imaging **23**(4), 501–509 (2004)

13. Zhang, J., Dashtbozorg, B., Bekkers, E., Pluim, J.P.W., Duits, R., ter Haar Romeny, B.M.: Robust retinal vessel segmentation via locally adaptive derivative frames in orientation scores. IEEE Trans. Med. Imaging **35**(12), 2631–2644 (2016)

14. Dashtbozorg, B., Mendonça, A.M., Campilho, A.: An automatic graph-based approach for artery/vein classification in retinal images. IEEE Trans. Image Process. **23**(3), 1073–1083 (2014)

15. Decencière, E., et al.: TeleOphta: machine learning and image processing methods for teleophthalmology. IRBM **34**(2), 196–203 (2013)

16. Vanschoren, J., Van Rijn, J.N., Bischl, B., Torgo, L.: OpenML: networked science in machine learning. ACM SIGKDD Explorations Newsletter **15**(2), 49–60 (2014)

Real Data Augmentation
for Medical Image Classification

Chuanhai Zhang[1]([⊠]), Wallapak Tavanapong[1], Johnny Wong[1],
Piet C. de Groen[2], and JungHwan Oh[3]

[1] Department of Computer Science, Iowa State University, Ames, IA, USA
{czhang89, tavanapo, wong}@iastate.edu
[2] Department of Medicine, University of Minnesota, Minneapolis, MN, USA
degroen@umn.edu
[3] Department of Computer Science and Engineering,
University of North Texas, Denton, TX, USA
Junghwan.Oh@unt.edu

Abstract. Many medical image classification tasks share a common unbalanced data problem. That is images of the target classes, e.g., certain types of diseases, only appear in a very small portion of the entire dataset. Nowadays, large collections of medical images are readily available. However, it is costly and may not even be feasible for medical experts to manually comb through a huge unlabeled dataset to obtain enough representative examples of the rare classes. In this paper, we propose a new method called Unified LF&SM to recommend most similar images for each class from a large unlabeled dataset for verification by medical experts and inclusion in the seed labeled dataset. Our real data augmentation significantly reduces expensive manual labeling time. In our experiments, Unified LF&SM performed best, selecting a high percentage of relevant images in its recommendation and achieving the best classification accuracy. It is easily extendable to other medical image classification problems.

Keywords: Real data augmentation · Unbalanced data · Image classification

1 Introduction

To use supervised machine learning in the medical domain, highly skilled expertise is required to create a training dataset with sufficient representative images for all the classes. Data imbalance is prevalent due to two major factors. For a given disease of interest, there are more healthy patients than unhealthy ones. For a given patient, typically there are more normal images than the abnormal ones. For instance, in a colonoscopic procedure, most frames showing normal colon mucosa compared to no frames or a few minutes of frames showing a polyp and a snare for polypectomy.

Traditional data augmentation is commonly used to address the data imbalance problem [1, 2]. This approach applies image processing operators such as translation, cropping, and rotation on images in the training dataset to create more images for the classes with fewer labeled samples. However, the limitation is that, depending on the parameters and image operators used, the generated samples may not represent image

© Springer International Publishing AG 2017
M.J. Cardoso et al. (Eds.): CVII-STENT/LABELS 2017, LNCS 10552, pp. 67–76, 2017.
DOI: 10.1007/978-3-319-67534-3_8

appearances in real data or the generated samples may be very similar to the existing images in the training dataset. Random data dropout addresses the data imbalance problem by randomly dropping out data of the class with many more examples (e.g., the normal class) [3]. However, this method does not increase the learning capability for the rare classes.

We investigate a different paradigm that selects images from a large unlabeled dataset and recommends them to the medical expert. We call this paradigm "real data augmentation" since the recommended images are from a real dataset. One naive real data augmentation method is to select images from the unlabeled dataset randomly without replacement and ask the medical expert to assign them class labels. This approach is time-consuming and costly to obtain enough representative examples of the rare target classes. On the other hand, a self-training method [4] applies a probabilistic classifier trained on the seed labeled dataset to predict the class of each unlabeled image and recommend for each class the images with the highest probabilities of belonging to that class. However, the low classification accuracy caused by the small training dataset likely results in incorrect recommendations. Some real data augmentation methods were introduced for text classification [5] and object recognition [6]. These methods use two steps. First, the feature representation is learned. Then, a fixed distance function, (e.g., the L2 distance, the cosine similarity), is used to retrieve relevant samples.

Our contribution in this paper is as follows. (1) We propose a new real data augmentation method called Unified Learning of Feature Representation and Similarity Matrix (Unified LF&SM) using a single deep Convolution Neural Network (CNN) trained on the seed labeled dataset. The method recommends top k similar images to the training images for each class to augment the seed dataset for that class. (2) We explore two more real data augmentation methods, the two-step method that learns feature representation first then learns the similarity matrix later and the method that learns only feature representation using a fixed similarity function. (3) We evaluated the effectiveness of the three methods and the self-training method. The effectiveness is in terms of the number of relevant images in the top k recommended images and the classification accuracy for the problem of 6-class classification of colonoscopy and upper endoscopy images. We found Unified LF&SM most effective among the four methods in our experiments.

2   Methods

We describe four methods for real data augmentation in this section. They differ in how feature representations are obtained and the recommendation algorithm to select unlabeled images. Let T be a labeled training image dataset, N_C be the number of classes desired for the classification problem, and N_j be the number of images in T belonging to a class j. Let U be an unlabeled dataset with a cardinality of N_s. Our goal is to recommend the set (R_j) of k most relevant images from U for each class j. We use CNN as our supervised deep learning classification algorithm. In this paper, we investigate the simplest recommendation algorithm, which recommends the top k most similar images for each class to improve the robustness of CNN. The higher the value of k is, the larger the variation in the recommended examples is. Note that even the most similar image is recommended, it is still useful since the image is from a different video never seen in the training set.

2.1   Data Augmentation Based on Probabilities (CNN + Probability)

After training a CNN classifier on T, we apply the classifier to each image I_i in $\mathcal{U}$ and obtain the corresponding value $p_{(i,j)}$ indicating the probability of the image I_i belonging to a class j using the soft-max function at the last layer of the CNN. Figure 1 shows the recommendation algorithm. The structure of the CNN we used is described in Sect. 3.1.

```
for j = 1,2,...,N_C
  for i = 1,2,...,N_S
    Compute p_(i,j) using the CNN classifier
  end for
  Sort p_(1:N_S, j) in descending order /* sort images based on probability */
  Assign top k images to the set R_j for the class j
end for
Return R_j for each class j
```

Fig. 1. Recommendation algorithm—"CNN + Probability"

2.2   Data Augmentation Based on Distance Function Learning (CNN + Bilinear)

We train a CNN classifier on the training dataset T. Then we extract the feature representation v_i for the image I_i using the trained CNN. Next, we apply OASIS [7] to learn a bilinear similarity function $S_W(v_i, v_j)$ in Eq. 1 that assigns higher similarity scores to images in the same class. Figure 2 shows our method based on the bilinear similarity function to find similar images.

```
for j = 1,2,...,N_C
  Compute the center of the feature vectors of all images of
  the class j in T: v̄ = Σ_{i=1}^{N_j} v_i/N_j
  for i = 1,2,...,N_S
    Compute v_i^T W v̄ as similarity score S_W(i,j)
  end for
  Sort S_W(1:N_S, j) in descending order /* sort images based on similarity score */
  Assign top k images to the set R_j for the class j
end for
Return R_j for each class j
```

Fig. 2. Recommendation algorithm—"CNN + Bilinear"

$$S_W(v_i, v_j) = v_i^T W v_j \tag{1}$$

2.3 Data Augmentation Based on Feature Learning (Triplet + L2)

We train Facenet triplet learning model [8] on the seed training dataset T that aims at learning an embedding (feature representation) function $\mathcal{F}(I_i)$, from an image I_i into its corresponding feature vector by minimizing the overall loss L calculated using Eq. 2. We want to achieve the goal that the squared distance between the image I_i and the image I_i^+ of the same class as I_i must be at least α smaller than the squared distance between the image I_i and image I_i^- of a different class as I_i as shown in Eq. 3. The second term $\lambda \sum_{\theta \in P} \theta^2$ in Eq. 2 is the regularization term [9] to prevent overfitting and obtain a smooth model. λ is the weight decay.

$$L = \sum_{i=1}^{N_\Gamma} \max\left(0, \left\|\mathcal{F}(I_i) - \mathcal{F}(I_i^+)\right\|_2^2 + \alpha - \left\|\mathcal{F}(I_i) - \mathcal{F}(I_i^-)\right\|_2^2\right) + \lambda \sum_{\theta \in P} \theta^2 \tag{2}$$

$$\left\|\mathcal{F}(I_i) - \mathcal{F}(I_i^+)\right\|_2^2 + \alpha < \left\|\mathcal{F}(I_i) - \mathcal{F}(I_i^-)\right\|_2^2, \forall (I_i, I_i^+, I_i^-) \in \Gamma \tag{3}$$

where α is an enforced margin between positive and negative pairs; P is the set of all parameters in $\mathcal{F}(I_i)$; I_i^+ (positive) is an image from the same class as I_i. I_i^- (negative) is an image from a different class as I_i. Γ is the set of all possible triplets in the training set and has cardinality N_Γ. Figure 3 shows our method based on the learned embedding function using the squared distance function (L2) to find similar images.

```
for j = 1, 2, ..., N_C
    Compute the center of the feature vectors of all images of
    the class j in T: v̄ = Σ_{i=1}^{N_j} F(I_i)/N_j
    for i = 1, 2, ..., N_S
        distance d(i, j) = ‖F(I_i) − v̄‖_2^2
    end for
    Sort d(1: N_S, j) in ascending order /* sort images based on L2 distance */
    Assign top k images to the set R_j for the class j
end for
Return R_j for each class j
```

Fig. 3. Recommendation algorithm—"Triplet + L2"

2.4 Unified Learning of Feature Representation and Similarity Matrix

We describe our proposed **U**nified **L**earning of **F**eature Representation and **S**imilarity **M**atrix (Unified LF&SM). Figure 4 shows the new model structure which is trained on the seed training dataset T. We aim at finding a similarity score model $S_{(\mathcal{F}, W)}(I_i, I_j)$, which is a pair of an embedding function $\mathcal{F}(I_i)$ mapping an image I_i into a feature vector and a bilinear similarity matrix W, such that the similarity score between the image I_i and the image I_i^+ of the same class as I_i must be at least α bigger than the similarity score between the image I_i and image I_i^- of a different class as I_i as shown in Eqs. 4 and 5.

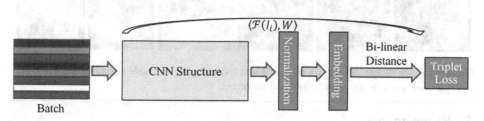

Fig. 4. The model consists of a batch input layer to a CNN followed by L2 normalization, which results in the embedding using the triplet loss based on the Bi-linear distance.

```
for j = 1,2,...,N_C
    Compute the center of the feature vectors of all images of
    the class j in T: v̄ = Σ_{i=1}^{N_j} F(I_i)/N_j
    for i = 1,2,...,N_S
        similarity score S_{(F,W)}(i,j) = F(I_i)^T W v̄
    end for
    Sort S_{(F,W)}(1:N_S,j) in descending order /* sort images based on similarity score */
    Assign top k images to the set R_j for the class j
end for
Return R_j for each class j
```

Fig. 5. Recommendation algorithm—"Unified LF&SM"

$$S_{(\mathcal{F},W)}\left(I_i, I_i^+\right) > S_{(\mathcal{F},W)}\left(I_i, I_i^-\right) + \alpha, \forall (I_i, I_i^+, I_i^-) \in \Gamma \tag{4}$$

$$S_{(\mathcal{F},W)}\left(I_i, I_j\right) = (\mathcal{F}(I_i))^T W \mathcal{F}(I_j) \tag{5}$$

We minimize the loss function as shown in Eqs. 6 and 7 to obtain the above mentioned similarity score model.

$$L = \sum_{i=1}^{N_\Gamma} l_{\mathcal{F},W}\left(I_i, I_i^+, I_i^-\right) + \lambda \sum_{\theta \in P} \theta^2 \tag{6}$$

$$= \sum_{i=1}^{N_\Gamma} \max\left(0, \alpha - S_{(\mathcal{F},W)}\left(I_i, I_i^+\right) + S_{(\mathcal{F},W)}\left(I_i, I_i^-\right)\right) + \lambda \sum_{\theta \in P} \theta^2 \tag{7}$$

where the definition of α, N_Γ, I_i^- and I_i^+ are the same as in Sect. 2.3; P is the set of all parameters in $\mathcal{F}(I_i)$ and W. Unlike the Facenet model that uses L2 distance and optimizes for the feature representation, the new model does joint optimization on both the feature representation and the similarity learning function. Figure 5 shows our recommendation algorithm using the learned similarity matrix and the learned feature representation to find unlabeled images similar to the training images for each class.

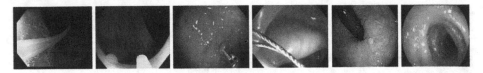

Fig. 6. Sample images for the six classes. From left to right: left cable body, right cable body, forceps head, snare head, retroflexion, and no object.

3 Experiments

To evaluate the performance of the four data augmentation methods, we selected two image classification problems in endoscopy video analysis: the instrument image detection [10] and the retroflexion image detection [11]. These two problems share a common unbalanced data problem; instrument images and retroflexion images are rare as the proportions of these images are very small as shown in Table 1. Figure 6 shows sample images for left cable body, right cable body, forceps head, snare head, retroflexion, and no object class for common endoscopy images without any of the aforementioned objects. We solve these two problems using one six-class CNN classifier.

Table 1. Average percentage of images belonging to each class calculated on the 25 training videos.

Class name	Ratio (%)
Left cable body	2.01
Right cable body	3.82
Forceps head	2.04
Snare head	1.51
Retroflexion	0.80
No object	89.8

Table 2. Our CNN structure. The input and output sizes are described in rows × cols × # nodes. The kernel is specified as rows × cols × #filters, stride.

Layer	Size-in	Size-out	Kernel
Conv1	$64 \times 64 \times 3$	$64 \times 64 \times 16$	$3 \times 3 \times 16,1$
Pool1	$64 \times 64 \times 16$	$32 \times 32 \times 16$	$2 \times 2 \times 16,2$
Conv2	$32 \times 32 \times 16$	$32 \times 32 \times 32$	$3 \times 3 \times 32,1$
Pool2	$32 \times 32 \times 32$	$16 \times 16 \times 32$	$2 \times 2 \times 32,2$
Conv3	$16 \times 16 \times 32$	$16 \times 16 \times 64$	$3 \times 3 \times 64,1$
Pool3	$16 \times 16 \times 64$	$8 \times 8 \times 64$	$2 \times 2 \times 64,2$
Conv4	$8 \times 8 \times 64$	$8 \times 8 \times 128$	$3 \times 3 \times 128,1$
Pool4	$8 \times 8 \times 128$	$4 \times 4 \times 128$	$2 \times 2 \times 128,2$
Conv5	$4 \times 4 \times 128$	$1 \times 1 \times 256$	$4 \times 4 \times 256,1$

Training dataset: We extracted and labeled one frame for every five frames from 25 de-identified full-length endoscopic videos of colonoscopy and upper endoscopy captured using Fujinon or Olympus scopes. Finally, we get a training set of 9300 images (1400 training images and 150 validation images for each class, $N_C = 6$). Table 1 shows the average percentage of images belonging to each class calculated on the 25 training videos.

Unlabeled dataset $\mathcal{U}$ consists of 600,000 unlabeled images ($N_s = 600,000$) from 228 endoscopic videos by automatically extracting one frame for every ten frames. Each unlabeled video is different from any training video.

Test dataset consists of 21000 images (3500 test images for each class) from 58 endoscopic videos by automatically extracting one frame for every five frames. Each test video is different from any training video and unlabeled video. The test dataset contains many rare-class images with quite different appearances (e.g., different instrument colors or shapes) from the training images.

3.1 Model Parameters

Considering the fact that only a small training set is available, we use a CNN structure which is similar to the VGG Net [12], but has much fewer parameters, as shown in Table 2. Our CNN models accept RGB images with the size of 64 × 64 pixels. These images are from resizing the raw endoscopic images. We implemented our CNN models using Python and Google's TensorFlow library [13]. When training the CNN classifiers described in Sects. 2.1 and 2.2, we set the batch size as 256 and the epoch number as 400. When training the CNN models described in Sects. 2.3 and 2.4, we set the enforced margin α as 0.2, the weight decay λ as 0.001, the epoch number as 200 (400 batches per epoch, 6 classes per batch, and 512 images by random selection per class). We learned the bilinear similarity function in Sect. 2.2 using the Matlab code provided by the author of OASIS and set the iteration number as 10^8. The feature vector of each image comes from the output of the "Conv5" in Table 2. To show the advantage of the proposed real data augmentation over the traditional data augmentation, we used KERAS [14] to apply rotation (0°–30°), shearing (0–0.01), translation (0–0.01), zooming (0–0.01), and whitening on each image in the seed training dataset and synthesized 5600 images for each class to expand the seed training dataset.

Table 3. Comparison of 6-class image classification performance for different models.

Method	Average recall	Average precision
Baseline	80.3%	80.8%
Traditional augmentation	83.2%	84.0%
CNN + Probability	84.4%	85.0%
CNN + Bilinear	85.8%	86.0%
Triplet + L2	88.9%	89.2%
Unified LF&SM	**89.3%**	**89.3%**

3.2 Performance Metrics and Comparison

3.2.1 Classification Performance

We trained the new CNN classifier by adding the new correctly recommended images ($k = 5000$) to the seed dataset for each recommendation model and computed the average recall and average precision on the six classes. When training the CNN classifier for each method, we used the same CNN structure, weight decay, and learning rate.

In Table 3, Baseline represents the CNN classifier trained on the seed dataset. Table 3 shows that we can get the best average recall and average precision when using the Unified LF&SM to do real data augmentation. Table 3 also shows that, compared to the Baseline, the Unified LF&SM improved the average recall and the average precision by 9% and 8.5%, respectively. Table 3 also shows that even the simple method of selecting top k similar images still outperforms the traditional data augmentation that is commonly used. This result shows that our real data augmentation method is very useful for improving the image classification accuracy. Although the classification performance between Triplet + L2 and Unified LF&SM is very close, we will see next that Unified LF&SM reduces the efforts of manual labeling the most.

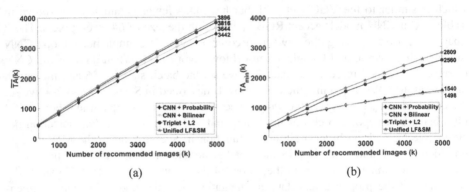

Fig. 7. (a)–(b) $\overline{TA}(k)$ and $TA_{min}(k)$ for the top k recommended images.

3.2.2 Efforts of Domain Experts

We define the number of true accepts (correct recommendations) in the top k recommended images for the class j as $TA(j,k)$. We define $\overline{TA}(k)$ as the average true accepts considering all classes for each k, a desired number of recommend images. We define $TA_{min}(k)$ as the number of true accepts for the class with the least correct recommendations among all the classes. We use the actual number instead of precision to reflect the medical experts' efforts to verify the recommended results.

$$\overline{TA}(k) = \sum_{j=1}^{N_c} TA(j,k)/N_c \quad TA_{min}(k) = \min_{1 \leq j \leq N_c} TA(j,k) \tag{8}$$

As shown in Fig. 7, the difference in true accepts increases as k increases. When k is small ($<=1000$), the difference in the correctness of the recommendation is small. As k becomes larger, the better technique makes more correct recommendations. Figure 7 also shows that Unified LF&SM outperforms the three other methods by recommending 80–454 more true accepts (average number) and recommending 249–1311 more true accepts (minimum number) for the top 5000 recommendations. Although the difference on classification performance between Triplet + L2 training and Unified LF&SM in Table 3 is very small, but Unified LF&SM reduces the manual labeling workload as shown in Fig. 7. Figure 7(b) shows that when comparing the minimum number of true accepts for all classes, Unified LF&SM and "Triplet + L2" show a much better result than "CNN + Bilinear" and "CNN + Probability." The explanation is that the two latter methods have the class "snare head" as the class with the least correct recommendations and recommended fewer relevant images for the class "snare head". One reason to explain the large performance difference is that the models using the triplet have many more training samples (N^3 in theory where N is the number of images in the training set) than those of the models using the single image input (only N) in the training process.

Assume we want to get k number of images belonging to the class j and the ratio of images belonging to the class j in the training video is r as shown in Table 1, then we estimate the number of images to be labeled using random selection as k/r in the fourth column of Table 4. For example, the estimated number is $202720 \approx 3061/(1.51\%)$ for the class "snare head". Table 4 shows that, to obtain the same number of true accepts for a rare target class, medical experts have to verify at least 26 ($130680/5000 \approx 26$) times the number of images if using random selection of unlabeled images compared to if using Unified LF&SM. With Unified LF&SM, medical experts spend far less time on annotating ground truth, and still give adequate representative images for the rare target class.

Table 4. Comparison of the number of images to be labeled using random selection and Unified LF&SM for each rare target class to obtain the same number of true accepts.

Class name	#True accepts	# Unified LF&SM	#Random selection
Left cable	4600	5000	228860
Right cable	4992	5000	130680
Forceps head	2809	5000	137700
Snare head	3061	5000	202720
Retroflexion	2923	5000	365380

3.3 Applicability to Other Types of Medical Images

Our Unified LF&SM automatically learns the image feature vector and the similarity matrix to recommend images when only given a small labelled image dataset. Therefore, the Unified LF&SM does not require specific domain knowledge on medical images and is easily extendable to other medical image classification problems.

4 Conclusion

We have presented and evaluated our Unified LF&SM with the goal to decrease the time needed for creating the training data by medical experts. We achieved this goal for the classification problems of instrument and retroflexion images. Our future work includes investigating a better recommendation algorithm, exploring active learning by repeatedly recommending images in iterations using the proposed Unified LF&SM, and extending the approach for object localization and temporal scene segmentation for medical image and video analysis.

References

1. Tajbakhsh, N., et al.: Convolutional neural networks for medical image analysis: full training or fine tuning? TMI **35**(5), 1299–1312 (2016)
2. Chatfield, K., et al.: Return of the devil in the details: delving deep into convolutional nets. arXiv preprint (2014). arXiv:1405.3531
3. Shin, H.C., et al.: Learning to read chest x-rays: recurrent neural cascade model for automated image annotation. In: CVPR, pp. 2497–2506 (2016)
4. Zhu, X.: Semi-supervised Learning Literature Survey (2005)
5. Lu, X., et al.: Enhancing text categorization with semantic-enriched representation and training data augmentation. JAMIA **13**(5), 526–535 (2006)
6. Xu, Z., et al.: Augmenting strong supervision using web data for fine-grained categorization. In: ICCV, pp. 2524–2532 (2015)
7. Chechik, G., et al.: Large scale online learning of image similarity through ranking. J. Mach. Learn. Res. **11**, 1109–1135 (2010)
8. Schroff, F., Kalenichenko, D., Philbin, J.: Facenet: a unified embedding for face recognition and clustering. In: CVPR, pp. 815–823 (2015)
9. Bishop, C.: Pattern Recognition and Machine Learning, pp. 144–146. Springer, New York (2007)
10. Zhang, C., et al.: Cable footprint history: spatio-temporal technique for instrument detection in gastrointestinal endoscopic procedures. In: IPCV, pp. 308–314 (2015)
11. Wang, Y., et al.: Near real-time retroflexion detection in colonoscopy. JBHI **17**(1), 143–152 (2013)
12. Simonyan, K., Zisserman, A.: Very deep convolutional networks for large-scale image recognition. arXiv preprint (2014). arXiv:1409.1556
13. Abadi, M., et al.: TensorFlow: large-scale machine learning on heterogeneous distributed systems. arXiv preprint (2016). arXiv:1603.04467
14. Chollet, F.: Keras. https://github.com/fchollet/keras

Detecting and Classifying Nuclei on a Budget

Joseph G. Jacobs[1,2]([✉]), Gabriel J. Brostow[2], Alex Freeman[3],
Daniel C. Alexander[1,2], and Eleftheria Panagiotaki[1,2]

[1] Centre for Medical Image Computing, University College London, London, UK
j.jacobs@cs.ucl.ac.uk
[2] Department of Computer Science, University College London, London, UK
[3] Department of Histopathology, University College London Hospitals
NHS Foundation Trust, University College London, London, UK

Abstract. The benefits of deep neural networks can be hard to realise in medical imaging tasks because training sample sizes are often modest. Pre-training on large data sets and subsequent transfer learning to specific tasks with limited labelled training data has proved a successful strategy in other domains. Here, we implement and test this idea for detecting and classifying nuclei in histology, important tasks that enable quantifiable characterisation of prostate cancer. We pre-train a convolutional neural network for nucleus detection on a large *colon* histology dataset, and examine the effects of fine-tuning this network with different amounts of *prostate* histology data. Results show promise for clinical translation. However, we find that transfer learning is not always a viable option when training deep neural networks for nucleus *classification*. As such, we also demonstrate that semi-supervised ladder networks are a suitable alternative for learning a nucleus classifier with limited data.

1 Introduction

Measures of cell nuclei show increasing promise for improving cancer characterization, providing useful diagnostic and prognostic information for different pathologies. For instance, the amount of different types of cells in prostate tissue (epithelial, fibroblast, etc.) strongly correlates to the Gleason grade of prostate cancer [3,5]. Lee et al. [7] show that nuclei orientation entropy in prostatectomies is a predictor of biochemical recurrence in cancer patients. However, such quantitative histological analysis is rarely used in clinical practice: manual nucleus detection and classification is *extremely* time consuming due to the high resolution of histological images, and the requisite expertise is also expensive. There is a critical need for computer-aided diagnosis tools for nuclei in histology.

Automatic nucleus detection is a well studied problem [1,6]. The current state-of-the-art systems use convolutional neural networks (CNNs) to perform spatial regression for predicting the location of nuclei [12,15]. Similarly, the best nucleus type classification methods also use CNNs. Sirinukunwattana et al. [12] use an ensemble of CNN predictions to classify images containing previously detected nuclei. Wang et al. [14] go a step further and train CNNs for simultaneous nucleus detection and classification in lung biopsies while Bayramoglu and

M.J. Cardoso et al. (Eds.): CVII-STENT/LABELS 2017, LNCS 10552, pp. 77–86, 2017.
DOI: 10.1007/978-3-319-67534-3_9

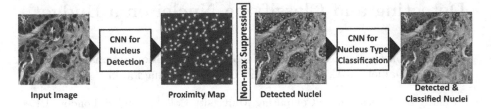

Fig. 1. Pipeline for detecting and classifying nuclei in histology.

Heikkilä [2] show that transfer learning from natural images is useful for improving both the training time and performance of nucleus classification CNNs. While these perform impressively, a limitation of CNNs is that they typically require fully supervised training with thousands of labelled nuclei to prevent overfitting. This can be a major barrier for entry within the medical community as the data needs to be labelled by expert clinicians, which makes producing large labelled datasets expensive, both in time and cost.

This paper examines methods for learning a prostate nucleus detector and classifier given modest amounts of labelled prostate nuclei data. Specifically, we explore the viability of transfer learning for prostate nucleus detection by fine-tuning CNNs pre-trained on colon data and semi-supervised learning with Γ-ladder networks for prostate nucleus classification. These methods attempt to exploit the availability of large amounts of data from other domains (transfer learning) and large amounts of unlabelled prostate data (semi-supervised learning) respectively. The following sections describe the detail of these methods (Sect. 2) and our experiments (Sect. 3).

2   Methods

This section describes the CNN models (Subsect. 2.1), the fine-tuning procedure used to perform transfer learning (Subsect. 2.2) and the ladder network architecture used for semi-supervised learning (Subsect. 2.3).

2.1   Detecting and Classifying Nuclei with CNNs

Nucleus Detection. Like [6,12,15] we formulate nucleus detection as a regression task as seen in Fig. 1. Given an input histology image, the nucleus detector predicts a function $d(x)$ that expresses the proximity of each pixel x to the nearest nucleus centroid. The local maxima in the resulting proximity map correspond to predicted nucleus centroids. We use the proximity function from [6]:

$$d(x) = \mathbb{I}\Big[D(x) \leq d_{\max}\Big]\left(e^{\alpha\left(1-\frac{D(x)}{d_{\max}}\right)} - 1\right) \tag{1}$$

where $\mathbb{I}[a]$ is an indicator function, $D(x)$ is the Euclidean distance from x to the nearest nucleus centroid while α and $d_{\max}$ control the height and radius of

Table 1. The fully convolutional network for nucleus detection.

#	Type	Filter size	Stride	Padding
1	Convolution	$7 \times 7 \times 3 \times 16$	1×1	3×3
2	ReLU			
3	Max pooling	3×3	1×1	1×1
4	Convolution	$5 \times 5 \times 16 \times 16$	1×1	2×2
5	ReLU			
6	Max pooling	3×3	1×1	1×1
7	Convolution	$5 \times 5 \times 16 \times 16$	1×1	2×2
8	ReLU			
9	Max pooling	3×3	1×1	1×1
10	Convolution	$11 \times 11 \times 16 \times 128$	1×1	5×5
11	ReLU			
12	Convolution	$1 \times 1 \times 128 \times 128$	1×1	0×0
13	ReLU			
14	Convolution	$1 \times 1 \times 128 \times 1$	1×1	0×0

peaks in $d(x)$. We introduce a novel fully convolutional network (FCN) architecture (Table 1) that performs inference on an entire image in a single pass. This significantly speeds up both training and test time compared to sliding window methods[1].

Nucleus Type Classifier. The nucleus type classifier is a standard multi-class classification CNN that takes as input a 27×27px nucleus patch and classifies it as either epithelial, inflammatory or miscellaneous. The network structure is the standard single patch predictor model described in [12].

2.2   Transfer Learning with CNNs

Unlike other machine learning methods, CNNs do not require hand-engineered input features. The convolutional layers in a CNN act as feature extractors that are learnt directly from data. However, this can be a major limitation as these convolutional filters need to be trained on large datasets to prevent overfitting. One way to avoid re-learning the convolutional filters for every task is by transfer learning. Instead of training a CNN from scratch, we begin with a model that is pre-trained on a separate, large dataset. This ensures that the model has useful convolutional filters when we begin training. The training procedure then fine-tunes these CNN weights for a particular task.

---

[1] It takes approximately 80 min to process a $107\,250 \times 103\,168$ whole-slide prostatectomy image on an NVIDIA GTX980 (incl. disk I/O), comparable to [16].

We examine the suitability of using transfer learning for reducing the amount of training data required to train both nucleus classifiers and detectors. For both tasks, we pre-train CNNs on a publicly available dataset of labelled colon nuclei [12] and fine-tune the entire CNN with varying amounts of prostate data. This allows investigation of the trade-off between the amount of labelled prostate training data and performance of nucleus detection/classification CNNs.

2.3   Semi-supervised Learning with Ladder Networks

Another method for reducing the amount of labelled training data required is by using a semi-supervised learning framework. Given a dataset of N labelled images and M unlabelled images where often $M \gg N$, semi-supervised learning frameworks attempt to learn classification models that exploit both the labelled and unlabelled images. In this instance, we explore the suitability of the ladder network architecture [11] for learning a nucleus classifier. Ladder networks turn a standard neural network into a semi-supervised model by treating it as the encoder in a denoising autoencoder.

A standard neural network is turned into a ladder network by (i) adding a decoder network to turn the network into an autoencoder and (ii) adding skip connections from every layer in the encoder to the corresponding layer in the decoder. During training, noise is added to the outputs of each layer in the encoder and the training objective is to minimise the weighted sum of the supervised cost function and the unsupervised cost functions[2]. A special case of ladder networks is the Γ-ladder network where we only consider the denoising cost in the top-most layer of decoder network (i.e. we set the denoising cost weights of all other decoder layers to zero). In our experiments, we use the Γ-ladder CNNs to perform semi-supervised learning of nucleus classifiers as they are faster to train and have fewer hyperparameters to adjust.

3   Results and Discussion

3.1   Experimental Setup

Dataset. All experiments were run on a dataset of H&E stained prostate biopsies collected from 34 cancer patients. The biopsies were digitised at $20\times$ magnification ($0.55\,\mu$m per pixel) with a Leica SCN400 slide scanner and we extracted 400 250×250px images. A histopathologist with over 10 years experience in genitourinary pathology (AF) dot annotated 16,562 nuclei in these images. 10,062 of these were also labelled with one of three nuclei type labels: 4212 epithelial, 1866 inflammatory (lymphocytes, plasma cells and macrophages) and 3984 miscellaneous (fibroblasts, blood vessel walls, nerves, etc.). We divided this data into three patient-stratified sets: 40% for training, 10% for validation and 50% for testing.

---

[2] The supervised objective is the cross entropy cost at the top of the encoder while the unsupervised objectives are the denoising mean squared errors at each decoder layer. We refer the reader to [11] for a more detailed description of ladder networks.

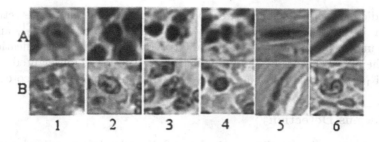

Fig. 2. Sample nuclei from the prostate (row A) and colon (row B) datasets. Columns 1 & 2 are epithelial nuclei, 3 & 4 are inflammatory nuclei and 5 & 6 are other miscellaneous nuclei.

For the fine-tuned models we pre-train the CNNs on a publicly available colon biopsy dataset [12]. The images are also H&E stained and digitised at 20× magnification. The dataset contains 29,756 dot annotated nuclei, with type labels for 22,444 nuclei: 7,722 epithelial, 6,971 inflammatory and 7,751 miscellaneous.

CNN Training. The CNN weights were randomly initialised from a normal distribution with mean 0 and standard deviation of 10^{-2}. The data was augmented with 90°, 180° and 270° rotations as well as flips along the horizontal and vertical axes. We trained the networks using stochastic gradient descent with Nesterov momentum [13] with a learning rate of 10^{-4} and minibatch sizes of 2 250 × 250px image patches for the nucleus detectors[3] and 128 27 × 27 nucleus patches for the nucleus classifiers. To prevent overfitting, the number of training epochs was determined independently for each network based on the value of the cost function on the held-out validation set. The optimal number of epochs ranged from as few as 20 training epochs for classification networks pre-trained on colon data to 5,000 training epochs for fully supervised classification CNNs trained using just 1% of labelled prostate training data. Other hyperparameters such as the unsupervised cost weight were similarly optimised on the held-out validation set independently for each network to prevent overfitting.

Evaluation Metrics. We quantify the performance of a model by measuring the number of true positives (TP), false positives (FP) and false negatives (FN) produced by the model. TPs, FPs and FNs are well defined for classification problems. For nucleus detection, we define a TP as a predicted centroid that falls within a 6px radius of the ground truth annotation. FPs are predictions that do not meet this criterion and FNs are ground truth annotations not associated

---

[3] We note that since the FCN performs dense prediction on an input image, training/testing with a single 250 × 250px image patch is equivalent to training/testing with 62,500 neighbouring patches using a patch-based method.

with predictions. Based on these, we report four metrics for nucleus detection: (i) precision, $P = \frac{TP}{TP+FP}$ (ii) recall, $R = \frac{TP}{TP+FN}$, (iii) F_1 score, $F_1 = \frac{2PR}{P+R}$ and (iv) the area under the precision-recall curve (AUPR). For nucleus classification, we report the overall accuracy, the individual class F_1 scores, unweighted average of class F_1 scores (macro F_1) and the weighted average of class F_1 scores.

3.2 Nucleus Detection

Table 2 compares the baseline method (a CNN trained from scratch with the given labelled images) against a fine-tuned CNN pre-trained with colon data. The precision, recall and F_1 scores reported on the table are for the point on the precision-recall curve with the highest F_1 score. The results show that fine-tuned CNNs consistently outperform the baseline method. Although the precision, recall and F_1 scores of the baseline methods are similar to that of the fine-tuned models, the more revealing metric is the AUPR. The fine-tuned CNNs have much higher AUPR than baseline CNNs. Using just 1% of labelled prostate data, the fine-tuned CNN AUPR is comparable to that of the baseline method that uses 100% of labelled data (Fig. 3). This indicates that the fine-tuned CNNs are more robust to the choice of the threshold parameter used to discard false positives. The results also suggest that the convolutional filters learnt with the colon data are generalisable to prostate data for this task.

Table 2. Precision, recall, F_1 score and AUPR for nucleus detectors trained with different amounts of labelled prostate images.

Labelled	Metrics	Baseline CNN	Fine-tuned CNN
1% 2 images	Precision	0.805 ± 0.002	$\mathbf{0.827 \pm 0.007}$
	Recall	0.862 ± 0.012	$\mathbf{0.873 \pm 0.004}$
	F_1 Score	0.833 ± 0.006	$\mathbf{0.849 \pm 0.003}$
	AUPR	0.866 ± 0.004	$\mathbf{0.896 \pm 0.001}$
3% 6 images	Precision	0.825 ± 0.005	$\mathbf{0.836 \pm 0.012}$
	Recall	0.863 ± 0.009	$\mathbf{0.872 \pm 0.015}$
	F_1 Score	0.844 ± 0.003	$\mathbf{0.853 \pm 0.001}$
	AUPR	0.877 ± 0.006	$\mathbf{0.899 \pm 0.005}$
5% 10 images	Precision	0.824 ± 0.007	$\mathbf{0.845 \pm 0.002}$
	Recall	$\mathbf{0.875 \pm 0.005}$	0.865 ± 0.003
	F_1 Score	0.849 ± 0.003	$\mathbf{0.855 \pm 0.002}$
	AUPR	0.885 ± 0.003	$\mathbf{0.901 \pm 0.001}$
100% 200 images	Precision	0.843 ± 0.013	$\mathbf{0.846 \pm 0.004}$
	Recall	$\mathbf{0.885 \pm 0.007}$	0.882 ± 0.004
	F_1 Score	$\mathbf{0.864 \pm 0.005}$	$\mathbf{0.864 \pm 0.003}$
	AUPR	0.910 ± 0.003	$\mathbf{0.911 \pm 0.004}$

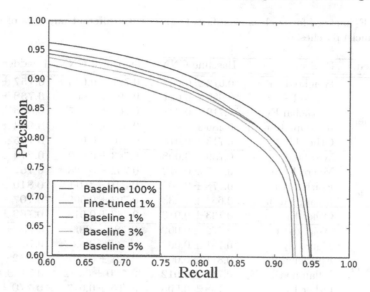

Fig. 3. Precision-recall curves for the baseline models and the 1% fine-tuned model.

3.3 Nucleus Classification

For nucleus classification, we compare our baseline method (a fully supervised CNN) against a fine-tuned CNN and a Γ-ladder CNN (Table 3). The results show that fine-tuning does not work very well when using 1% of labelled training data. Despite a 4–5% increase across the mean F_1 scores, we note that the scores have larger standard deviations compared to the baseline and Γ-ladder CNN, especially for inflammatory nuclei. The Γ-ladder CNN performs substantially better than the other two models across the different metrics using just 1% of the labelled data. The Γ-ladder CNN trained with 1% of labelled data even outperforms the baseline trained on 3% of labelled data on five of the six metrics.

We see a considerable jump in performance for the baseline and fine-tuned models when 3% of labelled data is used for training. While the Γ-ladder CNN improves as well and is still the best performing of the three models, the increase in performance is less substantial. Similarly, there is a marginal improvement in performance of all the three models as we increase the amount of labelled data to 5%. When using 100% of labelled data, we see identical performance for all models, with Γ-ladder CNNs performing marginally better than the other two.

The experiments indicate that Γ-ladder CNNs are the most robust of the three models. They perform well even when given a very small amount of labelled data and either matches or improves the performance of fully supervised and fine-tuned models when we increase the amount of labelled data. The large variation in inflammatory nucleus classification performance at 1% of labelled data could be explained by the small fraction of inflammatory nuclei in the prostate dataset compared to the other classes. However, as previously noted there is an even larger variation in inflammatory nucleus classification performance for the

Table 3. F_1 metrics for nucleus classifiers trained with different amounts of labelled prostate nuclei patches.

Labelled	F_1 Scores	Baseline CNN	Fine-tuned CNN	Γ-ladder CNN
1% 40 nuclei	Weighted F_1	0.672 ± 0.007	0.721 ± 0.043	$\mathbf{0.757 \pm 0.017}$
	Macro F_1	0.639 ± 0.021	0.695 ± 0.061	$\mathbf{0.738 \pm 0.019}$
	Epithelial F_1	0.719 ± 0.031	0.765 ± 0.027	$\mathbf{0.806 \pm 0.015}$
	Inflammation F_1	0.486 ± 0.089	0.574 ± 0.145	$\mathbf{0.654 \pm 0.034}$
	Other F_1	0.713 ± 0.018	0.746 ± 0.017	$\mathbf{0.755 \pm 0.014}$
3% 120 nuclei	Weighted F_1	0.739 ± 0.008	0.763 ± 0.010	$\mathbf{0.774 \pm 0.008}$
	Macro F_1	0.725 ± 0.012	0.752 ± 0.008	$\mathbf{0.762 \pm 0.010}$
	Epithelial F_1	0.778 ± 0.009	$\mathbf{0.810 \pm 0.007}$	$\mathbf{0.810 \pm 0.009}$
	Inflammation F_1	0.664 ± 0.033	0.703 ± 0.006	$\mathbf{0.707 \pm 0.018}$
	Other F_1	0.733 ± 0.013	0.743 ± 0.018	$\mathbf{0.769 \pm 0.006}$
5% 200 nuclei	Weighted F_1	0.772 ± 0.002	$\mathbf{0.780 \pm 0.009}$	0.779 ± 0.007
	Macro F_1	0.761 ± 0.003	$\mathbf{0.769 \pm 0.007}$	0.765 ± 0.008
	Epithelial F_1	0.811 ± 0.006	0.821 ± 0.007	$\mathbf{0.822 \pm 0.008}$
	Inflammation F_1	0.713 ± 0.012	$\mathbf{0.720 \pm 0.012}$	0.704 ± 0.019
	Other F_1	0.758 ± 0.003	0.765 ± 0.017	$\mathbf{0.770 \pm 0.009}$
100% ~4000 nuclei	Weighted F_1	0.831 ± 0.004	0.828 ± 0.002	$\mathbf{0.835 \pm 0.004}$
	Macro F_1	0.820 ± 0.005	0.819 ± 0.002	$\mathbf{0.825 \pm 0.004}$
	Epithelial F_1	0.868 ± 0.003	0.863 ± 0.002	$\mathbf{0.872 \pm 0.003}$
	Inflammation F_1	0.772 ± 0.006	0.775 ± 0.003	$\mathbf{0.778 \pm 0.011}$
	Other F_1	0.821 ± 0.006	0.818 ± 0.001	$\mathbf{0.824 \pm 0.003}$

fine-tuned CNN compared to the other models. This could potentially be explained by differences between the colon and prostate datasets. Inflammatory cells in the prostate dataset are mainly lymphocytes (Fig. 2, A3) while inflammatory cells in the colon are mainly macrophages (Fig. 2, B3) which are active and therefore look very similar to abnormal epithelial cells (Fig. 2, B2) with visible nucleoli.

4   Conclusions and Future Work

This paper adapts the general principles of transfer learning and semi-supervised learning for detecting and classifying cell nuclei on a budget. We demonstrate that transfer learning is suitable for learning nucleus detectors and classifiers given limited labelled data. However, it could potentially cause problems if there are biological differences in the tissue characteristics between the dataset used for pre-training and the dataset used for fine-tuning, as seen when attempting to learn a nucleus classifier with transfer learning. In this instance, we demonstrate that semi-supervised learning with Γ-ladder networks is a suitable alternative.

In future work, we will explore methods for including the full ladder network architecture, as well as histology from different organs and pathologies that could benefit from this application (e.g. breast cancer). Additionally, a limitation of ladder networks is that they have more hyperparameters to optimise compared to standard neural networks. As such, future work will explore adapting other semi-supervised learning for neural networks [8], possibly adding query selection [4].

Acknowledgments. We thank the EPSRC for funding EP's (EP/N021967/1), DA's (EP/M020533) and GB's (EP/K015664/1, EP/K503745/1) work on this topic, the UCL Department of Computer Science for JJ's studentship and the UCL Computer Science Cluster team.

References

1. Arteta, C., Lempitsky, V., Noble, J.A., Zisserman, A.: Learning to detect cells using non-overlapping extremal regions. In: Ayache, N., Delingette, H., Golland, P., Mori, K. (eds.) MICCAI 2012. LNCS, vol. 7510, pp. 348–356. Springer, Heidelberg (2012). doi:10.1007/978-3-642-33415-3_43
2. Bayramoglu, N., Heikkilä, J.: Transfer learning for cell nuclei classification in histopathology images. In: Hua, G., Jégou, H. (eds.) ECCV 2016. LNCS, vol. 9915, pp. 532 539. Springer, Cham (2016). doi:10.1007/978-3-319-49409-8_46
3. Chatterjee, A., Watson, G., Myint, E., Sved, P., McEntee, M., Bourne, R.M.: Changes in epithelium, stroma, and lumen space correlate more strongly with glea-son pattern and are stronger predictors of prostate ADC changes than cellularity metrics. Radiology **277**(3), 751–762 (2015)
4. Gal, Y., Islam, R., Ghahramani, Z.: Deep bayesian active learning with image data. In: NIPS Bayesian Deep Learning Workshop (2016)
5. Gorelick, L., Veksler, O., Gaed, M., Gómez, J.A., Moussa, M., Bauman, G.S., Fenster, A., Ward, A.D.: Prostate histopathology: learning tissue component his-tograms for cancer detection and classification. IEEE Trans. Med. Imaging **32**(10), 1804–1818 (2013)
6. Kainz, P., Urschler, M., Schulter, S., Wohlhart, P., Lepetit, V.: You should use regression to detect cells. In: Navab et al. [9], pp. 276–283
7. Lee, G., Ali, S., Veltri, R., Epstein, J.I., Christudass, C., Madabhushi, A.: Cell orientation entropy (COrE): predicting biochemical recurrence from prostate can-cer tissue microarrays. In: Mori, K., Sakuma, I., Sato, Y., Barillot, C., Navab, N. (eds.) MICCAI 2013. LNCS, vol. 8151, pp. 396–403. Springer, Heidelberg (2013). doi:10.1007/978-3-642-40760-4_50
8. Maaløe, L., Sønderby, C.K., Sønderby, S.K., Winther, O.: Auxiliary deep genera-tive models. In: Balcan, M., Weinberger, K.Q. (eds.) ICML 2016, Proceedings of Machine Learning Research, PMLR, pp. 1445–1453 (2016)
9. Navab, N., Hornegger, J., Wells, W.M., Frangi, A.F. (eds.): MICCAI 2015. LNCS, vol. 9351. Springer, Cham (2015). doi:10.1007/978-3-319-24553-9
10. Ourselin, S., Joskowicz, L., Sabuncu, M.R., Unal, G., Wells, W. (eds.): MICCAI 2016. LNCS, vol. 9901. Springer, Cham (2016)
11. Rasmus, A., Berglund, M., Honkala, M., Valpola, H., Raiko, T.: Semi-supervised learning with ladder networks. In: Cortes, C., Lawrence, N.D., Lee, D.D., Sugiyama, M., Garnett, R. (eds.) NIPS 2015, pp. 3546–3554. Curran Associates, Inc. (2015)
12. Sirinukunwattana, K., Raza, S.E.A., Tsang, Y.W., Snead, D.R.J., Cree, I.A., Rajpoot, N.M.: Locality sensitive deep learning for detection and classification of nuclei in routing colon cancer histology images. IEEE Trans. Med. Imaging **35**(5), 1196–1206 (2016)

13. Sutskever, I., Martens, J., Dahl, G., Hinton, G.: On the importance of initialization and momentum in deep learning. In: Dasgupta, S., McAllester, D. (eds.) ICML 2013, Proceedings of Machine Learning Research, PMLR, pp. 1139–1147 (2013)
14. Wang, S., Yao, J., Xu, Z., Huang, J.: Subtype cell detection with an accelerated deep convolution neural network. In: Ourselin et al. [10], pp. 640–648
15. Xie, Y., Xing, F., Kong, X., Su, H., Yang, L.: Beyond classification: structured regression for robust cell detection using convolutional neural network. In: Navab et al. [9], pp. 358–365
16. Xu, Z., Huang, J.: Detecting 10,000 cells in one second. In: Ourselin et al. [10], pp. 676–684

Towards an Efficient Way of Building Annotated Medical Image Collections for Big Data Studies

Yaniv Gur[✉], Mehdi Moradi, Hakan Bulu, Yufan Guo,
Colin Compas, and Tanveer Syeda-Mahmood

IBM Almaden Research Center, San Jose, CA 95120, USA
guryaniv@us.ibm.com

Abstract. Annotating large collections of medical images is essential for building robust image analysis pipelines for different applications, such as disease detection. This process involves expert input, which is costly and time consuming. *Semiautomatic labeling* and *expert sourcing* can speed up the process of building such collections. In this work we report innovations in both of these areas. Firstly, we have developed an algorithm inspired by active learning and self training that significantly reduces the number of annotated training images needed to achieve a given level of accuracy on a classifier. This is an iterative process of labeling, training a classifier, and testing that requires a small set of labeled images at the start, complemented with human labeling of difficult test cases at each iteration. Secondly, we have built a platform for large scale management and indexing of data and users, as well as for creating and assigning tasks such as labeling and contouring for big data medical imaging studies. This is a web-based platform and provides the tooling for both researchers and annotators, all within a simple dynamic user interface. Our annotation platform also streamlines the process of iteratively training and labeling in algorithms such as active learning/self training described here. In this paper, we demonstrate that the combination of the platform and the proposed algorithm significantly reduces the workload involved in building a large collection of labeled cardiac echo images.

1 Introduction

Over the last few years machine learning has found its way to many real-world applications. In certain tasks, it has enabled machine performance at or even above human level. However, to build robust and accurate machine learning solutions, large amounts of data need to be curated and labeled. While in many applications, such as image and speech recognition, large collections of labeled data can be easily obtained through crowd-sourcing over the Web, in the medical domain the situation is different. Although it is becoming clear that machine learning can aid clinicians to provide accurate diagnosis faster than before, the penetration of machine learning into the medical field has been hampered due to lack of high-quality labeled data. Since medical data is collected in the course

© Springer International Publishing AG 2017
M.J. Cardoso et al. (Eds.): CVII-STENT/LABELS 2017, LNCS 10552, pp. 87–95, 2017.
DOI: 10.1007/978-3-319-67534-3_10

of routine clinical practice and cannot leave secure networks due to privacy regulations, its availability is limited. In addition to that, medical data needs to be labeled by experts, but expert resources are scarce and costly. Some of these problems were tackled in [2,8] through expert and crowd-sourcing in the context of computer-assisted minimally-invasive surgery (MIS) and image modality detection. Other solutions have been proposed in the form of utilizing accompanying text sources to establish weak preliminary labels for the data [3].

In this paper, we take a general approach for expert-sourcing and introduce two complementary solutions to address the problem of labeling large collections of medical images. Firstly, we have developed a semi-supervised algorithm to reduce the number of expert-labeled samples needed to achieve a certain level of classification accuracy. This solution combines *active learning* [7] and *self training* [9]. Regardless of the classifier of choice, our algorithm improves the efficiency of data preparation.

Secondly, we built a web-based platform for user and data management that allows contouring and labeling of anonymized data through remote browsers, while the data remains at the clinical repository. This platform can be deployed on any server that stores medical data, and allows researchers to log in and create collections, labeling/contouring task templates, and assign them to users. Medical images are stored in a database structure that allows search and retrieval across labels and patient attributes for building and managing training and testing sets for machine learning.

We describe these two contributions in the context of two different experiments. In the first experiment, we use a convolutional neural network (CNN) for automatic labeling of ultrasound images for mode. In the second example, we use a support vector machine (SVM) to classify patients for presence and severity of aortic stenosis based on automatically extracted archival features. We show that one can significantly reduce the amount of data needed to be labeled by clinicians without compromising the accuracy, by implementing the proposed algorithm of semi-automatic labeling using our platform.

2   Semi-automatic Labeling

Active Learning is a semi-supervised approach in machine learning that addresses the problem of labeling big datasets while reducing manual labeling effort. It is based on an iterative process of training, prediction, and samples selection for manual labeling [7]. In active learning only manually labeled data is used to train a classifier. Self-training is another approach in which a classifier is trained on classifier-labeled data. In this section, we introduce an algorithm that is based on these two approaches and uses all the available data to achieve high classifier accuracy while dramatically reducing manual labeling effort. The platform introduced in Sect. 3 is an inseparable part of this process, as it streamlines the labeling process and makes it very efficient.

Our starting point is a small set of labeled images $\mathcal{D}_0 = \{(x_i, y_i) | i = 1, \ldots, N_0\}$ where N_0 is the number of samples, and y_i is the label of sample x_i. We first train a classifier using $\mathcal{D}_0$ and produce a model M_0. The model accuracy is tested in all the steps on a separate and fixed validation set, $\mathcal{V}$. We have a larger dataset of N_1 unlabeled samples, $\mathcal{S}_1 = \{(x_i, ?)|i = 1, \ldots, N_1\}$. We want to build an improved classifier using this dataset, without needing to manually label all the samples.

We start by automatically labeling $\mathcal{S}_1$ using M_0, where the outcome is a label $M_0(x_i) = y_i$ and a vector of class likelihoods per sample:

$$P(y_i|x_i) = \{P(y_i = 0|x_i), P(y_i = 1|x_i), \ldots, P(y_i = k - 1|x_i)\}, \qquad (1)$$

where k is the number of classes in the problem. Then we select a subset of samples for manual annotation by looking at the class likelihoods. All the samples with the largest class likelihood below a threshold $t \in (0, 1)$, that is, $max(P(y_i|x_i)) < t$, are considered as "hard cases" and selected for manual labeling, while labels with a class likelihood above the threshold are accepted as correct labels. For each of the hard cases, the predicted label is presented to an annotator on our annotation platform (Sect. 3), to accept or change. Once the manual labeling is completed, all the labels are combined to form a fully labeled set $\mathcal{S}_1$. Then, we create a new training set $\mathcal{D}_1 = \mathcal{D}_0 \cup \mathcal{S}_1$ and produce a learned model M_1, which is used to label a new set of unlabeled samples $\mathcal{S}_2$.

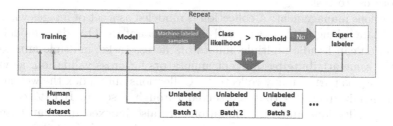

Fig. 1. The proposed algorithm for semi-automatic labeling based on our web-based annotation platform.

This process of labeling new sets in a semi-automatic fashion followed by re-training is repeated every time more data becomes available, or until the classifier reaches a desired accuracy on the validation set. See Fig. 1 for an overall description of this methodology. In experiments performed here, we divided all the available data into batches, and iterated the active learning cycle on the batches while monitoring the performance on an independent validation set. The validation set needs to be composed carefully by including equally distributed representatives from all the classes in the problem. Note that this approach is not specific to one classifier or another, as long as the classifier in hand provides class likelihood measures.

3 Web-Based Expert Sourcing of Image Annotations

In this section, we introduce the system we have developed for labeling and annotation of medical images on the web. The system addresses two problems in labeling large collections of medical images. It allows the efficient use of limited resources through expert sourcing. Secondly, it solves data and user management issues, allowing multiple annotators for a project, multiple annotations per image, and the ability to index and search across collections and annotations. The system provides the tooling for different annotation tasks, from image level labeling to object contouring, and is built with three design criteria in mind: flexibility of user interface in adding new features; scalability across image, tasks, users and tools dimensions; search capabilities across all labels, users, and task templates through indexing. In fact the main distinguishing factor of this system compared to some of the previous efforts in annotation through web browser such as [5] is an extensive machinery for data and user management that allows for streamlined use of data in machine learning algorithms, such as the active learning/self training process described in the previous section.

The platform is comprised of a user interface supported by three main backend modules:

1. User management: Provides the tools needed to register users in a database, control access to specific images and collections. Information about the annotators' expertise is also registered to allow for algorithmic matching of annotators to tasks.
2. Collections management: A collection is modeled as a set of images with their meta data, along with a task, and list of annotators. Our data model for a collection can handle multiple annotators across tasks, multiple annotations for the same attribute by different annotators for cross-validation, as well as one image as part of many collections. Collections only index the web address of anonymized images that are served through a secure HIPPA-compliant server. Collections and the annotations are also indexed in a database that allows search and retrieval across different image and label attributes such as mode, modality/specialty, and annotated clinical features.
3. Annotations management: Supports all the operations of defining annotation tasks, assigning annotators to collections based on their expertise, and tracking work progress by providing annotation completeness reports. The task and assignments per collection are also stored in the collections database. The process of task and collection assignment to annotators is done by authorized administrators, who have access to the image archive and the user database. User interfaces are built to support all these operations.

The flexibility of task building is obtained through a toolkit that allows a user to build a template. The template defines the type of task (such as contouring, labeling, measurement recording) and also the tools needed for performing the task. The user interface automatically interprets the template and shows the right tools and forms with the assigned collection of images. An example is shown in Fig. 2. In the example, users are expected to mark keypoint and draw a number of contours. The main features of the UI are described in Fig. 2.

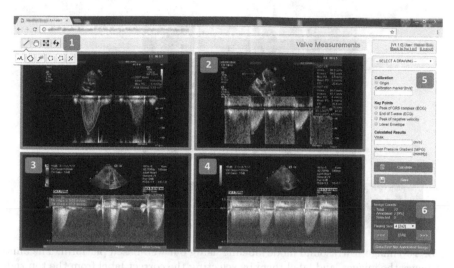

Fig. 2. User interface of our web-based annotation tool. This page is preceded by a user login, and task desktop for users. Toolbar (1) provides some common drawing tools with zooming and panning abilities. Green frames (2) indicate the annotated images. Blue frame (3) indicates the selected image. Red frame (4) indicate the image which has not been annotated yet. Annotation template (5) is used to set and save the annotation values and is supported by a task-specific template generating pipeline. Statistical frame (6) gives some key information to the user about status of the annotation task. Such as, number of total and annotated image counts and allows the user to navigate through the entire collection, or change the arrangement/number of images on page. (Color figure online)

4 Combining the Platform and Algorithm: Use Cases

In this section we demonstrate the use of the proposed algorithm and the developed platform on two use cases with different classifiers. The first example is built upon a convolutional neural network (CNN), while the second is built upon a support vector machine (SVM) classifier.

4.1 Mode Labeling in Cardiac Echo

In a cardiac echo exam, sonographers collect images of a variety of modes. Ultrasound mode in not always recorded in the DICOM header, but it needs to be detected for further analysis by systems that perform archival analysis of medical images such as [6]. The first use case described here is the task of building a convolutional neural network that classifies a given image in one of six possible modes. These are B-Mode, M-Mode, PW-Doppler, CW-Doppler, Color-Doppler, text-panels (Fig. 3). We started with a dataset of 980 images labeled by clinicians. This dataset was used to generate the initial learned model by training AlexNet [1] after reducing the number of network outputs to 6. The network was

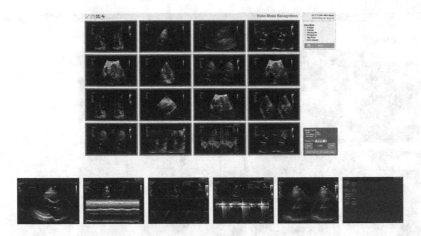

Fig. 3. Top image: Ultrasound mode labeling using our web-based platform. The annotator views the images, and label them by selecting the correct label from the top right menu and saving. Bottom image: The 6 classes in our problem. From left to right: B-mode, M-mode, PW-Doppler, CW-Doppler. Color-Doppler, and text-panel.

trained for 30 epochs with a batch size of 128 images, and was validated on a dataset of 3502 samples pre-labeled by clinicians.

4.2   Disease/Healthy Labels for Cardiac Echo Images

A second experiment was performed for the task of classifying patients for the presence of aortic stenosis, based on noisy measurements of maximum blood flow velocity and pressure gradient through the aortic valve, extracted from archival sources and automatic analysis of CW Doppler images. In our experiment, the described annotation platform was used for clinicians to examine CW Doppler images and label them for presence of aortic stenosis as the ground truth label for the patient. The classifier used in this experiment was a binary SVM, trained on a nine dimensional feature vector similar to the one described in [6]. 900 cases where available for the training phase of this experiment, along with an additional 100 cases solely used for testing. The SVM model was initially trained on 5 cases and data was added in batches of size 20.

5   Results

5.1   Ultrasound Mode Classification

The measured accuracy of the initial network trained on 980 manually labeled samples was 85.6% when tested on the independent validation set. We performed 4 iterations of semi-automatic labeling on equal size datasets consisting of 2060 images each. In each iteration we followed the steps described in Sect. 2. That is, we automatically labeled one batch of 2060 images using the model produced in the previous iteration. Then, we selected for manual labeling the samples with class likelihood of less than 0.9, and accepted the labels with likelihood above that threshold. Manual labeling was performed using our web-based platform where the images were organized in single label collections based on the network prediction. This way of organizing the data helped make manual labeling more efficient, as the annotator could quickly go through the images and relabel only the misclassified ones. After all the misclassification of hard cases were corrected, we formed a new training set by combining the new labeled samples (both hard cases and network-labeled cases) with the training set from the previous iteration, and retrained the network. This process was repeated until all 4 datasets were labeled. As shown in Fig. 4, after retraining with the first set of semi-automatically labeled samples, the classifier reached an accuracy of 97.4% that stabilized at 98% after the third labeling iteration. Moreover, the number of samples selected by the class likelihood criterion for manual labeling dropped dramatically from around 36% (771 samples) at the first iteration, to around 4% (85 samples) at the last iteration. Thus, by using this approach we reduced the labeling workload by a factor of 25 without compromising the accuracy. For reference, we compared the likelihood-based sampling strategy to random sampling at a constant rate of 25%. Our strategy outperformed random sampling and converged to a higher classifier accuracy with less manual labeling effort.

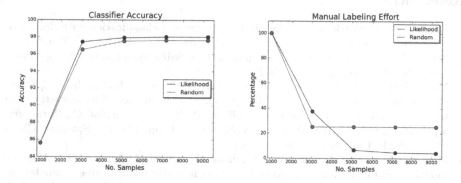

Fig. 4. Semi-automatic labeling with likelihood-based sampling vs. random sampling. Left figure: The CNN model accuracy as a function of the number of training samples. In random sampling the classifier accuracy converged to 97.6% vs. 98% in our approach. Right figure: The percentage of manually labeled samples in each iteration based on our selection criterion. The manual labeling rate using likelihood dropped from 100% in the initial set to only 4%.

5.2 Aortic Stenosis Detection

In the second experiment, the initial accuracy of stenosis detection for the classifier was 72%. We witnessed that after reaching 200 training samples, the classification accuracy saturated at 93%. We compared this trend with labeling and adding training data randomly without considering class likelihoods produced by the classifier. The same level of accuracy was achieved only after all 900 samples were labeled and included in training. In other words, the proposed algorithm reduced the labeling effort by 78%.

6 Conclusions

In this paper we introduced two innovations to address the problem of annotating large collections of medical images. We introduced an iterative semi-automatic image annotation approach that uses the web-based platform to reduce manual labeling effort by using a trained classifier. We demonstrated this approach on ultrasound mode labeling and achieved a classifier accuracy of 98% while reducing the manual labeling effort to 4% of an unlabeled samples set. We also introduced a web-based platform for expert sourcing of annotation tasks. This is built upon a comprehensive system for users, image collections, and annotations management to streamline machine learning studies of the type described here. Note that the algorithm and the platform described here are not limited to image labeling. For example, one can use a classifier like U-Net [4] to perform segmentation, and use our platform for expert feedback on selected samples before retraining the classifier. This and other use cases are currently under study.

References

1. Krizhevsky, A., Sutskever, I., Hinton, G.E.: Imagenet classification with deep convolutional neural networks. In: Pereira, F., Burges, C.J.C., Bottou, L., Weinberger, K.Q. (eds.) Advances in Neural Information Processing Systems, vol. 25, pp. 1097–1105. Curran Associates, Inc. (2012)
2. Maier-Hein, L., Mersmann, S., Kondermann, D., Bodenstedt, S., Sanchez, A., Stock, C., Kenngott, H.G., Eisenmann, M., Speidel, S.: Can masses of non-experts train highly accurate image classifiers? In: Golland, P., Hata, N., Barillot, C., Hornegger, J., Howe, R. (eds.) MICCAI 2014. LNCS, vol. 8674, pp. 438–445. Springer, Cham (2014). doi:10.1007/978-3-319-10470-6_55
3. Moradi, M., Guo, Y., Gur, Y., Negahdar, M., Syeda-Mahmood, T.: A cross-modality neural network transform for semi-automatic medical image annotation. In: Ourselin, S., Joskowicz, L., Sabuncu, M.R., Unal, G., Wells, W. (eds.) MICCAI 2016. LNCS, vol. 9901, pp. 300–307. Springer, Cham (2016). doi:10.1007/978-3-319-46723-8_35
4. Ronneberger, O., Fischer, P., Brox, T.: U-Net: convolutional networks for biomedical image segmentation. In: Navab, N., Hornegger, J., Wells, W.M., Frangi, A.F. (eds.) MICCAI 2015. LNCS, vol. 9351, pp. 234–241. Springer, Cham (2015). doi:10.1007/978-3-319-24574-4_28
5. Rubin, D.L., Willrett, D., O'Connor, M.J., Hage, C., Kurtz, C., Moreira, D.A.: Automated tracking of quantitative assessments of tumor burden in clinical trials. Translational Oncol. **7**, 300–307 (2014)
6. Syeda-Mahmood, T., Guo, Y., Moradi, M., Beymer, D., Rajan, D., Cao, Y., Gur, Y., Negahdar, M.: Identifying patients at risk for aortic stenosis through learning from multimodal data. In: Ourselin, S., Joskowicz, L., Sabuncu, M.R., Unal, G., Wells, W. (eds.) MICCAI 2016. LNCS, vol. 9902, pp. 238–245. Springer, Cham (2016). doi:10.1007/978-3-319-46726-9_28

7. Tong, S.: Active learning: theory and applications. Ph.D. thesis, Stanford University, August 2001
8. Vajda, S., You, D., Antani, S.K., Thoma, G.R.: Label the many with a few: semi-automatic medical image modality discovery in a large image collection. In: 2014 IEEE Symposium on Computational Intelligence in Healthcare and e-health (CICARE), pp. 167–173, December 2014
9. Zhu, X.: Semi-supervised learning literature survey. Technical report (2006)

Crowdsourcing Labels for Pathological Patterns in CT Lung Scans: Can Non-experts Contribute Expert-Quality Ground Truth?

Alison Q. O'Neil[1]($\boxtimes$), John T. Murchison[2], Edwin J.R. van Beek[3], and Keith A. Goatman[1]

[1] Toshiba Medical Visualization Systems Ltd., Edinburgh, UK
alison.j.oneil@gmail.com
[2] Royal Infirmary of Edinburgh, Edinburgh, UK
[3] Clinical Research Imaging Centre, University of Edinburgh, Edinburgh, UK

Abstract. This paper investigates what quality of ground truth might be obtained when crowdsourcing specialist medical imaging ground truth from non-experts. Following basic tuition, 34 volunteer participants independently delineated regions belonging to 7 pathological patterns in 20 scans according to expert-provided pattern labels. Participants' annotations were compared to a set of reference annotations using Dice similarity coefficient (DSC), and found to range between 0.41 and 0.77. The reference repeatability was 0.81. Analysis of prior imaging experience, annotation behaviour, scan ordering and time spent showed that only the last was correlated with annotation quality. Multiple observers combined by voxelwise majority vote outperformed a single observer, matching the reference repeatability for 5 of 7 patterns. In conclusion, crowdsourcing from non-experts yields acceptable quality ground truth, given sufficient expert task supervision and a sufficient number of observers per scan.

1 Introduction

Crowdsourcing is gaining in popularity as a method for sourcing labels for the very large amounts of data required to train machine learning algorithms [7]. Previous experiments have shown that it is possible to use non-experts for cheaply and readily crowdsourcing medical imaging ground truth [3,14], perhaps using gamification [1,11], at least for reasonably straightforward problems.

This paper investigates whether it is feasible to commission non-experts to undertake a relatively specialist imaging annotation task — that of recognising and segmenting the pathological patterns which are seen in interstitial lung disease. To this end, a toy exercise was designed in which participants were recruited to annotate the *same* representative set of twenty scan slices. In order to render the task accessible to the layperson, we restricted it to be one of annotation rather than diagnosis. Each scan slice was provided with expert labels indicating the presence of the main patterns to be labelled, and participants were asked to annotate regions belonging to these patterns. These labels are usually noted

© Springer International Publishing AG 2017
M.J. Cardoso et al. (Eds.): CVII-STENT/LABELS 2017, LNCS 10552, pp. 96–105, 2017.
DOI: 10.1007/978-3-319-67534-3_11

in a radiology report; thus the objective was for the routine expert diagnosis to direct the non-expert in the rather time-consuming work of delineating the pathological regions. To assess performance, we quantitatively and qualitatively compared the annotations to those of an expert medical researcher (A.O.) and two experienced radiologists (J.M. and E.v.B.) respectively.

The contributions of this paper are as follows:

- To demonstrate how a specialist medical imaging ground truth task may be simplified such that a non-expert (given some basic training) performs comparably to an expert.
- To analyse which factors are predictive of good performance.
- To demonstrate how (and how many) non-expert observers should be assigned and combined for each scan in a real world crowdsourcing task, in order to improve label robustness.
- To provide practical recommendations for how this task might be better conducted in future.

2 Methodology

2.1 Ground Truth for Interstitial Lung Disease

Identification of the presence, volume and distribution of different pathological patterns is helpful for the diagnosis and prognosis of interstitial lung disease [8]. Training machine learning algorithms to recognise and segment such patterns requires large amounts of labelled data. Thus, for this paper, the ground truth exercise was to label regions representing each of the common lung disease patterns: *consolidation, emphysema, ground glass opacity (GGO), ground glass opacity+reticulation, honeycombing, micronodules,* and *reticulation.* This is the same labelling system as used by Anthimopoulos *et al.* [2] for the same publicly available data [4], but with the addition of an emphysema class. Examples of these patterns are shown in Fig. 1.

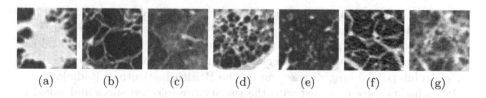

(a)   (b)   (c)   (d)   (e)   (f)   (g)

Fig. 1. Pathological lung patterns (a) *Consolidation* (b) *Emphysema* (c) *GGO* (d) *GGO+Reticulation* (e) *Honeycombing* (f) *Micronodules* (g) *Reticulation*

2.2 Data

Twenty computed tomography (CT) scan slices were selected from twenty different subjects in the MedGift ILD database [4]. The slices were chosen to span the range of disease labels, and each was labelled with one or two key patterns to be annotated by participants. Table 1 shows the pattern labels and medical diagnosis of each scan.

Table 1. Scan diagnoses (3 unknown) and patterns to label (C = *Consolidation*, E = *Emphysema*, G = *GGO*, GR = *GGO+Reticulation*, H = *Honeycombing*, M = *Micronodules*, R = *Reticulation*)

N	Diagnosis	Labels	N	Diagnosis	Labels
1	Idiopathic pulmonary fibrosis	E	11	Miliary tuberculosis	C, M
2	Idiopathic pulmonary fibrosis	H	12	Pulmonary Fibrosis	GR
3	Hypersensitivity pneumonitis	G, GR	13	Hypersensitivity pneumonitis	G
4	Miliary tuberculosis	M	14	–	H
5	–	E	15	Chronic eosinophilic pneumonia	R
6	Pulmonary fibrosis	R	16	Pulmonary tuberculosis	C
7	–	C	17	Hypersensitivity pneumonitis	R, GR
8	Cryptogenic organizing pneumonia	C, G	18	Hypersensitivity pneumonitis	G
9	Hypersensitivity pneumonitis	R, GR	19	Pulmonary fibrosis	E, GR
10	Hypersensitivity pneumonitis	H	20	Pulmonary fibrosis	H

2.3   Recruitment of Participants

The exercise was completed by 34 volunteers from a company which makes medical imaging software. The participants have a variety of roles and levels of expertise, including junior scientists and software engineers, senior managers, and clinical experts. Entry and exit questionnaires were completed by all the participants. The entry questions were designed to ascertain each participant's level of experience, and the factors motivating their participation. The exit questionnaire gathered feedback on participants' experience of the exercise, and suggestions for improvement.

2.4   Annotation Task

Prior to the annotation task, all participants received a one-hour long tutorial on interstitial lung disease and the patterns of interest (based on the Fleischner Society Glossary of Terms for Thoracic Imaging [5]), given by a biomedical sciences graduate (A.O.) who had recently attended a one-day hands-on training course on interstitial lung disease run by the British Institute of Radiology.

Participants were provided with the twenty pre-selected slices and asked to annotate patterns belonging to provided labels. Each participant annotated the images in a random order, to allow measurement of any training effect over the course of annotating the scans. Annotations were created using a tool that allowed users to draw polygonal regions of interest (ROIs) and assign a pattern class label to each ROI. The task was expected to take approximately two hours to complete. The use of online resources such as *Radiology Assistant* and *Google* was allowed and even encouraged, although collaboration between participants was prohibited.

3   Results

3.1   Evaluation of Non-expert Versus Expert Performance

Each annotation was scored by comparison to those of the reference annotator (A.O.) using Dice Similarity Score (DSC). The overall DSC was computed for each participant by weighting scans equally, and weighting patterns equally within a scan. Per-pattern DSC metrics were calculated for each participant by averaging over all examples of a pattern. In addition, the reference annotator repeated the annotations 10 days later to assess repeatability (the overall repeatability DSC was 0.806). Figure 2 summarises the results.

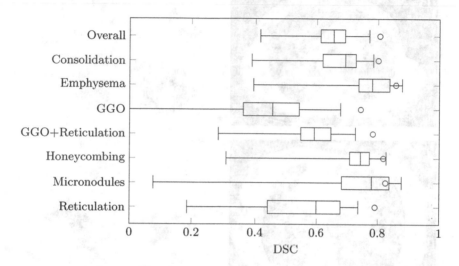

Fig. 2. The box plots indicate the median, upper and lower quartiles, and minimum and maximum DSC compared to the reference. The circles indicate the reference repeat scores.

There is clear variation in performance between classes, showing that some were more straightforward than others. It was known in advance that the distinction between e.g. *GGO, GGO+Reticulation,* and *Reticulation* might be open to interpretation. Also, there were a few cases of mistaken identity, with participants labelling vessels (pulmonary vessels and aorta) as pathology.

Following the exercise, interviews were held with two experienced pulmonary radiologists (J.M. and E.v.B.), who confirmed the veracity of the provided labels, and annotated the images with some obvious examples of each pattern. Figure 3 shows some qualitative results of four interesting cases, showing the radiologist and reference annotations overlaid on the results of the crowd.

It can be seen that for A (*Emphysema*) and B (*GGO*) in Fig. 3, the range of variation of the crowd is comparable to the agreement (or disagreement) between the two radiologists. In each case, one radiologist is more sensitive and the other

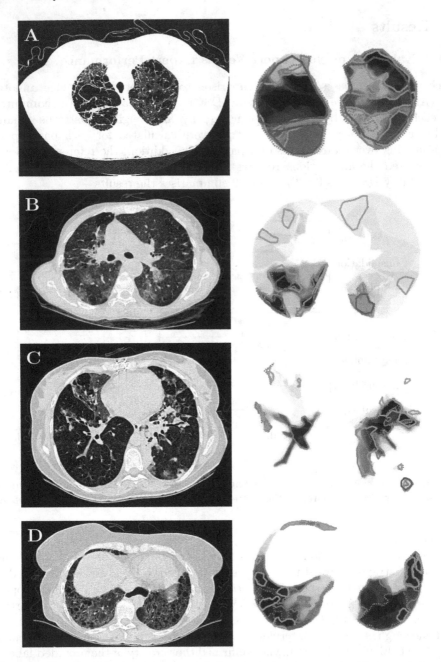

Fig. 3. Some example results: (A) Emphysema (B) GGO (C) Consolidation (D) Honeycombing. Scan slices are shown on the left and annotations are shown on the right. The greyscale background is proportional to the number of participants who annotated the label i.e. white = no annotations and black = all 34 annotations. The reference results are shown in magenta (dotted line for the repeat). The radiologists' annotations are shown in blue and green. (Color figure online)

more specific for the given pattern, and the crowd approximately ranges between the two.

Examples C and D illustrate where improvements could be made. In C (consolidation), it is difficult to distinguish vessels from consolidation. It can be seen that the radiologists were cautious with their labelling compared with the reference, who outlined both vessel and consolidation where they were adjacent and therefore not separable. The crowd generally followed the philosophy of the reference, but some of the crowd confused what is definitely vessel with consolidation. In D (honeycombing), both radiologists were stricter on the definition of honeycombing than the reference, and both raised the differential diagnosis with bronchiectasis. Honeycombing and bronchiectasis lie on a spectrum [12], and the bronchiectasis label was not included in our labelling system.

In summary, it was observed that in many cases the variability of the crowd matched the variability between the two radiologists, and this variability was reflective of underlying ambiguity in the pattern definition — or the ambiguity of the boundary between patterns such as *GGO* versus *GGO+reticulation*. However, in future the whole volume should be provided to the annotator rather than single slices, such that vessels can be better tracked and distinguished from consolidation (with appropriate teaching examples). We should also consider adding further labels such as bronchiectasis and fibrosis (fibrosis not illustrated here).

3.2 Factors Predicting Performance

None of the participants had specific prior experience of interstitial lung disease images. However, it was predicted that there may be a correlation between prior imaging experience and performance, particularly if insufficient training was provided for the task. Participants rated their level of experience with medical imaging data, from level 0 (little to none), to level 4 (clinical researcher). Figure 4 shows a plot of performance versus experience level. There is no significant correlation, suggesting that adequate guidance was provided for this task. Further, it was hypothesised that a training effect might be observed, however no correlation was measured between the scan ordering (randomised between participants) and each participant's performance.

Conversely, there is a weak correlation between the time spent on the task and performance (see Fig. 4). The times shown are self-reported estimates. It is likely that those participants who performed better took time to do more research and/or took more care with their annotations. Visible annotation behaviour (number of regions, number of polygon vertices, rate of polygon vertices) was also analysed and found to exhibit no correlation with performance.

3.3 Crowdtruthing in the Real World: Assigning and Combining Multiple Observers

The previous results have shown the range in annotation quality between observers. It is likely that more consistent results could be achieved by combining annotation results from multiple observers, and this is true also of expert

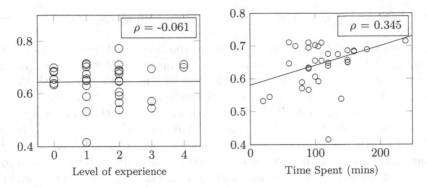

Fig. 4. Factors predicting performance. Level of expertise and time spent are plotted against DSC compared to the reference. Correlation coefficients are shown (Spearman's rank and Pearson's for the first and second plots respectively).

annotations, since human error or variations in pattern interpretation might be identified and corrected. In a real world crowdsourcing exercise, some questions would thus arise. How many observers should be assigned to each scan? How are their annotations best combined to give an annotation of predictable and reasonable quality?

To investigate this, different odd numbers of observers between one and fifteen were combined using majority vote at each voxel. For each number of observers, 200 combinations were randomly drawn from the 34 annotations, after omitting the few cases where the annotation was zero i.e. the participant had forgotten or was unable to label the key pattern. As in earlier DSC computations, the problem is simplistically treated as binary (i.e. a one-vs-all approach taken when evaluating each pattern), even where more than one pattern was labelled in a scan. The graphs in Fig. 5 show the median, minimum and maximum values, both overall and for each pattern, averaged across the twenty scans.

In summary, multiple observers give a better result than a single observer. The median increases and the range in DSC metrics narrows increasingly as more observers are added, with little improvement beyond the $k = 9$ observer. Note that the minimum, maximum and median converge at the limit of $n = 34$ observers, where there is just one possible combination of observers. For 5 of 7 patterns, the median DSC matches the repeat DSC and the range converges whilst $k \ll n$, showing that when sufficient observers are combined, the limit of accuracy is reached. For *GGO* and *GGO+Reticulation*, combination of multiple observers does not bring the crowd into agreement with the reference, suggesting that observers generally had a different idea to the reference for where the threshold between ground glass opacity and healthy tissue lies. STAPLE [15] methods were also tried (results not shown), initialised using both uniform (0.99999) and learnt rater sensitivities and specificities (learnt from the first ten scans and applied to the second ten), and STAPLE gave worse results than the majority vote. This is in line with what other authors have found [9,10].

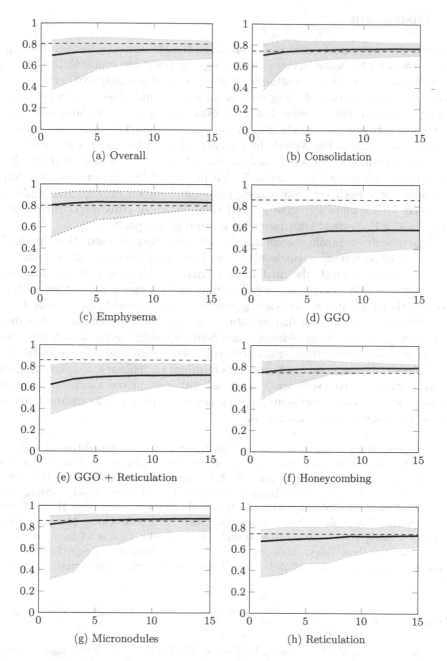

Fig. 5. Graphs showing the number of observers (x-axis) versus the reference DSC (y-axis) for the consensus (combined) annotation, for different pathological patterns. The solid lines indicate the median and the grey shading indicates the span from minimum to maximum (figures are the *mean* minimum, median and maximum across all scans). The dashed lines indicate the reference repeatability score.

4   Discussion

Overall, the crowd performed well relative to the reference segmentations, with some observers for some patterns matching the reference repeatability. Where there was variation, this was often indicative of genuine ambiguity between patterns. The greater range of disagreement for e.g. ground glass opacity compared to emphysema in this exercise has been observed by other authors measuring agreement between radiologists [13]. In fact, the combined annotations displayed as greyscale values in Fig. 3 could be interpreted as probabilities associated with the respective labels, and even used as soft labels for a machine learning algorithm in line with the "dark matter" idea promoted by Hinton *et al.* [6]. Note that agreement both between non-experts and between radiologists would be increased with a more stringent ground truth protocol (this might involve e.g. prescribing a Hounsfield Unit range for ground glass opacity).

Experiments regarding combination of observers showed that multiple observers outperformed a single observer. For many patterns, when sufficient observers are combined, the median DSC matches the reference repeatability DSC and the DSC range converges around the reference repeatability DSC, showing that the limit of accuracy is reached. Improvements as discussed earlier (additional teaching for distinguishing normal anatomy such as vessels from pathology, provision of three-dimensional context, additions to the labelling system, a more stringent ground truth protocol), should both raise the repeatability DSC and reduce the number of observers required to achieve a consistent result.

In conclusion, given sufficient expert task supervision and a sufficient number of observers per scan, crowdsourcing with non-experts can yield ground truth fit for use in image analysis algorithms.

Acknowledgements. Many thanks to Phil Tolland who developed the software for the ground truth collection tool, and to all of the employees at Toshiba Medical Visualization Systems who took part in this study: Allan Barklie, Erin Beveridge, Antony Brown, Gerald Chau, Alasdair Corbett, Ross Davies, Matt Daykin, Ben Docherty, Venkatesh Gaddam, Keith Goatman, Marta Guarisco, Joseph Henry, Corné Hoogendoorn, Pia Kullik, Aneta Lisowska, Steve Magness, Craig Matear, James Matthews, Chris McGough, Haritha Miryala, Brian Mohr, Costas Plakas, Ian Poole, Marco Razeto, Faye Riley, Matt Shepherd, Simeon Skopalik, Andy Smout, Ken Sutherland, Paul Thomson, Phil Tolland, John Tough, Aidan Wellington and Gavin Wheeler.

References

1. Albarqouni, S., Matl, S., Baust, M., Navab, N., Demirci, S.: Playsourcing: a novel concept for knowledge creation in biomedical research. In: Carneiro, G., et al. (eds.) LABELS/DLMIA -2016. LNCS, vol. 10008, pp. 269–277. Springer, Cham (2016). doi:10.1007/978-3-319-46976-8_28
2. Anthimopoulos, M., Christodoulidis, S., Ebner, L., Christe, A., Mougiakakou, S.: Lung pattern classification for interstitial lung diseases using a deep convolutional neural network. IEEE Trans. Med. Imaging **35**(5), 1207–1216 (2016)

3. Cheplygina, V., Perez-Rovira, A., Kuo, W., Tiddens, H.A.W.M., de Bruijne, M.: Early experiences with crowdsourcing airway annotations in chest CT. In: Carneiro, G., et al. (eds.) LABELS/DLMIA -2016. LNCS, vol. 10008, pp. 209–218. Springer, Cham (2016). doi:10.1007/978-3-319-46976-8_22
4. Depeursinge, A., Vargas, A., Platon, A., Geissbuhler, A., Poletti, P.A., Müller, H.: Building a reference multimedia database for interstitial lung diseases. Comput. Med. Imaging Graph. **36**(3), 227–238 (2012)
5. Hansell, D.M., Bankier, A.A., MacMahon, H., McLoud, T.C., Müller, N.L., Remy, J.: Fleischner society: glossary of terms for thoracic imaging. Radiology **246**(3), 697–722 (2008)
6. Hinton, G., Vinyals, O., Dean, J.: Distilling the knowledge in a neural network. In: Neural Information Processing Systems (2014)
7. Hossain, M., Kauranen, I.: Crowdsourcing: a comprehensive literature review. Strateg. Outsourcing Int. J. **8**(1), 1753–8297 (2015)
8. Humphries, S.M., Yagihashi, K., Huckleberry, J., Rho, B.H., Schroeder, J.D., Strand, M., Schwarz, M.I., Flaherty, K.R., Kazerooni, E.A., van Beek, E.J.R., Lynch, D.A.: Idiopathic pulmonary fibrosis: data-driven textural analysis of extent of fibrosis at baseline and 15-month follow-up. Radiology **5**, 161177 (2017)
9. Langerak, T.R., van der Heide, U.A., Kotte, A.N., Viergever, M.A., van Vulpen, M., Pluim, J.P.: Label fusion in atlas-based segmentation using a selective and iterative method for performance level estimation (SIMPLE). IEEE Trans. Med. Imaging **29**(12), 2000–2008 (2010)
10. Van Leemput, K., Sabuncu, M.R.: A cautionary analysis of STAPLE using direct inference of segmentation truth. In: Golland, P., Hata, N., Barillot, C., Hornegger, J., Howe, R. (eds.) MICCAI 2014. LNCS, vol. 8673, pp. 398–406. Springer, Cham (2014). doi:10.1007/978-3-319-10404-1_50
11. Luengo-Oroz, M.A., Arranz, A., Frean, J.: Crowdsourcing malaria parasite quantification: an online game for analyzing images of infected thick blood smears. J. Med. Internet Res. **14**(6), e167 (2012)
12. Piciucchi, S., Tomassetti, S., Ravaglia, C., Gurioli, C., Gurioli, C., Dubini, A., Carloni, A., Chilosi, M., Colby, T.V., Poletti, V.: From traction bronchiectasis to honeycombing in idiopathic pulmonary fibrosis: a spectrum of bronchiolar remodeling also in radiology? BMC Pulm. Med. **16**(1), 87 (2016)
13. Salisbury, M.L., Lynch, D.A., van Beek, E.J.R., Kazerooni, E.A., Guo, J., Xia, M., Murray, S., Anstrom, K.A., Yow, E., Martinez, F.J., Hoffman, E.A., Flaherty, K.R.: Idiopathic pulmonary fibrosis: the association between the adaptive multiple features method and fibrosis outcomes. Am. J. Respir. Crit. Care Med. **195**(7), 921–929 (2017)
14. Schlesinger, D., Jug, F., Myers, G., Rother, C., Kainmuller, D.: Crowdsourcing image segmentation with aSTAPLE. arXiv (2017)
15. Warfield, S.K., Zhou, K.H., Wells, W.M.: Simultaneous truth and performance level estimation (STAPLE): an algorithm for the validation of image segmentation. IEEE Trans. Med. Imaging **23**(7), 903–921 (2004)

Expected Exponential Loss for Gaze-Based Video and Volume Ground Truth Annotation

Laurent Lejeune[1], Mario Christoudias[2], and Raphael Sznitman[1(✉)]

[1] University of Bern, Bern, Switzerland
raphael.sznitman@artorg.unibe.ch
[2] Weather Analytics, Washington, DC, USA

Abstract. Many recent machine learning approaches used in medical imaging are highly reliant on large amounts of image and ground truth data. In the context of object segmentation, pixel-wise annotations are extremely expensive to collect, especially in video and 3D volumes. To reduce this annotation burden, we propose a novel framework to allow annotators to simply observe the object to segment and record where they have looked at with a \$200 eye gaze tracker. Our method then estimates pixel-wise probabilities for the presence of the object throughout the sequence from which we train a classifier in semi-supervised setting using a novel Expected Exponential loss function. We show that our framework provides superior performances on a wide range of medical image settings compared to existing strategies and that our method can be combined with current crowd-sourcing paradigms as well.

1 Introduction

Ground truth annotations play a critical role in the development of machine learning methods in medical imaging. Indeed, advances in deep learning strategies, coupled with the advent of image data in medicine have greatly improved performances for tasks such as structure detection and anatomical segmentation across most imaging modalities (*e.g.* MRI, CT, Endoscopy, Microscopy) [1,2]. Yet the process of acquiring ground truth data or annotations remains laborious and challenging, especially in video and 3D image data such as those depicted in Fig. 1.

To mitigate manual annotation dependence, semi- and unsupervised methods have been key research areas to reduce the overall annotation burden placed on domain experts (*e.g.* radiologist, biologist, surgeon etc.). Most notably, Active Learning (AL) [3,4], Transfer Learning (TL) [5,6] and Crowd-Sourcing (CS) [7,8] provide frameworks for learning with either limited or noisy ground truth data and have been applied to a larger number of applications. Yet in AL domain experts are still necessary to actively provide ground truth data, sequentially or in batch. Similarly, CS relies on manual annotators to follow carefully crafted labeling tasks in order to leverage non-experts, which produces highly variable ground truth quality [8].

© Springer International Publishing AG 2017
M.J. Cardoso et al. (Eds.): CVII-STENT/LABELS 2017, LNCS 10552, pp. 106–115, 2017.
DOI: 10.1007/978-3-319-67534-3_12

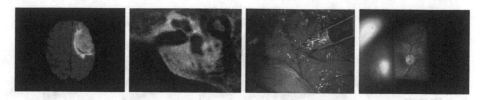

Fig. 1. Examples of volume and video data with a structure to annotate. Left to right: Brain tumor (3D-MRI), cochlea (3D-CT); surgical instrument (video endoscopy); optic disc (video microscope). Green contours highlight ideal ground truth regions. (Color figure online)

Alternatively, Vilariño et al. [9] used an eye gaze tracker to annotate polyps in video colonoscopy. In their approach an expert passively viewed a video and stared at polyps. From these, they trained an SVM classifier to label the sequence, treating regions around each gaze location as positives and the rest of the image domain as negative samples. As we show in our experiments however, this approach is limited to detecting objects of fixed size and does not extend well to pixel-wise segmentation tasks. Also related is the work in [10] which mapped out regions of interest using a gaze tracker on individual frames observed for extended periods of time. More recently, the work of [11] is closely related to our setting, with the important distinction that our data is viewed in one pass and applied to video and volumetric data.

To overcome this limitation, we propose a novel framework to produce pixel-wise segmentation for an object present in a volume (or video sequence) using gaze observations collected from a \$200 off-the-shelf gaze tracker. Assuming a single target is present throughout the image data, we cast our problem as a semi-supervised problem where samples are either labeled as positive (gazed image locations) or unknown (the rest of the image data which could be positive or negative). To learn in this regime, we introduce a new Expected Exponential loss function that can be used within a traditional gradient boosting framework. In particular, the expectation is taken with respect to the unknown labels, requiring a label probability estimate. We describe how to estimate these with a novel strategy and show that our approach not only provides superior performances over existing methods in a variety of medical imaging modalities (*i.e.* laparoscopy, microscopy, CT and MRI) but can be used in a crowd-sourcing context as well.

2   Gaze-Based Pixel-Wise Annotation

Our goal is to produce a pixel-wise segmentation of a specific structure of interest located in a video or in a volume (*i.e.* we treat a volume as a video sequence). To do this, we ask a domain expert to watch and follow the structure throughout the sequence. While viewing the sequence, we track the persons eye gaze by means of a commercially available eye gaze tracker. In our setting, this provides a single

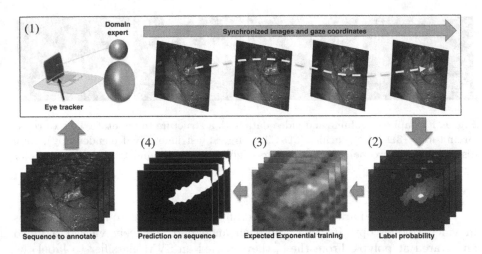

Fig. 2. Example Gaze-based annotating. A surgical instrument must be annotated in a sequence. (1) A domain expert watches the sequences and has their gaze collected during the viewing. (2) Our method then estimates object likelihoods over the sequence and (3) we then train a classifier with an Expected Exponential loss function using a subset of the image data. (4) The classifier is then used to evaluate the remainder of the sequence.

gaze location for each viewed image and we assume the observer is compliant in the task.

To produce ground truth annotations, we cast this problem as a binary semi-supervised machine learning problem, where one must determine a pixel-wise segmentation of the structure of interest in each of the images using only the sequence itself and the gaze locations. We assume that gaze locations correspond to the structure and propose a novel Expected Exponential loss function that explicitly takes into account that some labels are known while others are not. This loss leverages probability estimates regarding the unknown labels and we present a strategy to estimate these effectively. Note that, we do not focus on learning a function that generalizes to other similar sequences, but one that annotates the given sequence as well as possible.

For a given image sequence, our approach is organized as follows and is illustrated in Fig. 2: (1) the expert views the sequence and 2D gaze locations are collected; (2) we estimate the label probability by using the image data and the gaze information; (3) we then train a gradient boosted classifier with our proposed loss on a subset of the image data; (4) using the trained classifier, we predict the remainder of the image data. We will detail these steps in the following sections but first define some notation used throughout this paper.

Notation: Let an image sequence (or volume) be denoted $\mathcal{I} = [I_0, \ldots, I_T]$ and let $\mathcal{G} = \{g_t\}_{t=0}^T$ such that $g_t \in \mathbb{R}^2$ is a 2D gaze pixel location in I_t. While we ideally would like a pixel-wise segmentation, we choose to decompose each image using a temporal superpixel strategy [12] and operate at a superpixel level instead. We thus let I_t be described by the set of non-overlapping superpixels $S_t = \{S_t^n\}_{n=0}^{N_t}$ and define the set of all superpixels across all images as $S = \{S_t\}_{t=0}^{T}$. We denote the set $\mathcal{P} = \{S_t^n | g_t \subset S_t^n, t = 0, \ldots, T, n = 0, \ldots N_t\}$ as all superpixels observed and the rest as $\mathcal{U} = S \setminus \mathcal{P}$. We associate with each S_t^n a binary random variable $Y_t^n \in \{-1, 1\} = \mathcal{Y}$, such that $Y_t^n = 1$ if S_t^n is part of the object and -1 otherwise. In particular, we defined Y_n as a Bernoulli random variable, $Y_t^n \sim Ber(\epsilon_{S_t^n}), \epsilon_{S_t^n} \in (0, 1)$. Note that for superpixels observed by gaze $S_t^n \in \mathcal{P}$, we consider these as part of the object and let $Y_t^n = 1$ with $\epsilon_{S_t^n} = 1$.

3   Learning with an Expected Exponential Loss

Expected Exponential Loss (EEL): Our goal is to train a prediction function, $f : S \to \mathcal{Y}$ that takes into account observed superpixels as well as the unobserved ones. To do this we propose the following EEL function

$$\mathcal{E}\mathcal{E} = \mathbb{E}^Y \left[\sum_{S \in \{\mathcal{P}, \mathcal{U}\}} e^{-f(S)Y} \right] \tag{1}$$

where the expectation is taken with respect to all Ys. By linearity of expectation and the fact that labeled superpixels have no uncertainty in their label, we can rewrite the loss for all superpixels as

$$\mathcal{E}\mathcal{E} = \sum_{S \in \mathcal{P}} e^{-f(S)} + \sum_{S \in \mathcal{U}} \left(\epsilon_S e^{-f(S)Y} + (1 - \epsilon_S) e^{f(S)Y} \right) \tag{2}$$

Note that this Eq. (2) is a generalization of the Exponential Loss (EL) [13]. In the case where labels are known, the loss is the same as the traditional loss as the expectation is superfluous. For unknown samples, the value of ϵ_S weighs the impact of the superpixels. For instance, if ϵ_S is close to 0.5 then the sample does not affect the loss. Conversely values of ϵ_S close to 1 (or 0) will strongly impact the loss.

Implementation: We implemented the above EEL within a traditional Gradient Boosting classifier [13], by regressing to the residual given by the derivate of Eq. (2). For all experiments, we used stumps as weak learners, a shrinkage factor of 1 and the line search was replaced by a constant weight of 1. The weak learner stumps operate on features extracted from the center of the superpixel. In particular, we used generic Overfeat features [14] which provide a rich characterization of a region and its context (e.g. 4086 sized feature vector).

During training we used all superpixels in $\mathcal{P}$ and used 10% of those in $\mathcal{U}$. A total of 50 boosting rounds was performed in all cases. To predict segmentations for the entire volume, we predicted the remaining 90% of superpixels in $\mathcal{U}$.

4   Probability Estimation for Unknown Labels

To estimate ϵ_S in Eq. (2), we take inspiration from the Label Propagation method [15], which uses a limited number of positive and negative samples to iteratively propagate labels to unobserved samples. In our setting however, we only propagate positive samples to unlabeled samples using the gaze information as well as pixel motion estimation to constrain the probability diffusion.

We let $P_0 = [p_0, \ldots, p_N]$ be a vector of initial probabilities for all superpixels in a given image, where $p_n = P(Y = 1|\mathcal{P})$ is the probability that superpixel S_n is part of the object. In practice, we estimate p_n by computing a gaze dependent Lab color model using all gaze locations and assessing how likely a superpixel S_n is part of the object. That is, we compute

$$p_n = \max_{S \in \mathcal{P}} \mathcal{N}(S_n | \mu_S, \Sigma_S), \tag{3}$$

where $\mathcal{N}$ is a Gaussian distribution such that μ_S and Σ_S are the color mean and covariance of pixels in a superpixel S that was gazed at. For superpixels that were gazed at, their probability is fixed at 1. To propagate probabilities, we also define a $N \times N$ affinity matrix, denoted W with values

$$w_{ij} = \exp(-|\theta_i - \theta_j|_2/2\sigma_a^2)\exp(-|C(S_i) - C(S_j)|_2/2\sigma_d^2), \tag{4}$$

where for superpixel S_i, $C(S_i)$ is its center and θ_i is its average gradient orientation. In cases where S_i and S_j are separated by more than τ pixels, $w_{ij} = 0$. σ_a and σ_d are model parameters reflecting the variance in angle difference and the impact of neighboring superpixels, respectively.

Propagation can then be computed iteratively by solving

$$P_{m+1} = \alpha \Omega P_m + (1 - \alpha)P_0, \tag{5}$$

where $\alpha \in (0, 1)$ is a diffusion parameter, D is a diagonal matrix with entries $d_{ii} = \sum_j w_{ij}$ and $\Omega = D^{-1/2}WD^{-1/2}$. Figure 3 shows the initial P_0, the associated optical flow regions and the final propagated probability for a given image. While the original method described in [15] hinged on a minimum of one positive and one negative sample to prove the existence of a closed form convergence solution, the same cannot be said of the current setting where no negative samples are known. For this reason, we iterate a total of 10 times and then use the estimates for the ϵ_S values in Eq. (2). This value was experimentally determined and shown to perform well for a number of image sequences (see Sect. 5). The process is repeated for all frames in the sequence.

Note that the probability estimate is computed from a single gaze sequence and the corresponding image data. As such, if more than one domain expert viewed the same sequence, as it is the case in Crowd-Sourcing tasks, this process can be repeated for each observer and averaged over all observers. In our experiments, we show that doing so brings increased performances over that given by a single observer.

5   Experiments

To evaluate the performance of our method we compare it to the method presented in Vilariño et al. [9]. We also show how the EEL approach compares with

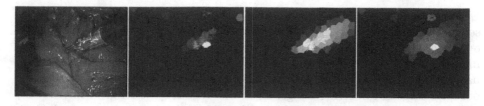

Fig. 3. Probability propagation. Left to right: original image with the gaze location highlighted in green; Initial P_0 estimate from the gaze-based color model; Image regions with high optical flow; Estimated probability after propagation. Dark blue regions depict low probability while warmer regions correspond to higher probabilities. (Color figure online)

that of using ϵ_S estimates only (see Sect. 4), as well using ϵ_S, with a traditional EL when binarizing the labels using a fixed threshold $\epsilon_S = 0.5$. The following parameters were kept constant: $\alpha = 0.95, \sigma_a = 0.5, \sigma_d = 50, \tau = 50$ and the superpixel size was set to match $1°$ on the viewing monitor.

We evaluated each of the above mentioned methods on 4 very different image sequences (see Fig. 1 for examples): (1) a 3D brain MRI containing a tumor to annotate from the BRATS challenge [16] consisting of 73 slices, (2) a 30 frame surgical video sequence from the MICCAI EndoVision challenge[1] where a surgical instrument must be annotated, (3) a 95-slice 3D CT scan where a cochlea must be annotated and (4) a slit-lamp video recording (195 frames) of a human retina where the optic disk must be segmented. Pixel-wise annotated ground truth on all frames of each sequence was either available or produced by a domain expert. In all sequences, one and only one object is present throughout the sequence.

Our method was implemented in MATLAB and takes roughly 30 min to segment a 30 frame volume with 720×576 sized frames, of which the bulk of time is used to compute temporal superpixels and training our classifier. Even though real-time requirements are not necessary in this application, we believe this computation time could be reduced with an improved implementation

Gaze locations were collected with an Eye Tribe Tracker (Copenhagen, Denmark) which provide $1°$ degree tracking accuracy. To collect gaze locations, a computer monitor and the tracker was placed roughly 1 m from the experts face. Device-specific calibration was performed before all recordings (*i.e.* a 2-minute long procedure done once before each viewing). 2D gaze locations were collected and mapped to the viewed image content using the manufacturers API. Domain experts were instructed to stare at the target and avoid looking at non-object image regions. Once each sequence was observed, the different methods inferred the object throughout the entire image data.

Results – Annotation accuracy: Table 1 reports the Area Under the Curve (AUC) and the F-score performances of each method applied to each dataset. In general, we report that the proposed combined label estimation and

---

[1] Endoscopic vision challenge: https://endovis.grand-challenge.org.

EEL function provide the highest AUC and F-score values across the tested sequences. Figure 4 visually depicts example frames from each sequence and the outcome of each method, as well as the ground truth. To generate these binary images, a %5 false positive threshold was applied (*i.e.* threshold was determined using the ground truth). One can see that in cases where the object to segment occupies large areas of the image, as is the case for the surgical instrument, both the traditional loss approach and that of [9] do not perform as well since they treat significant portions of the background as positive samples during their respective learning phases.

Table 1. Area under the curve (AUC) and performances for each approach on each dataset. highlight maximum values in bold.

Dataset	Metric	Vilarino et al. [9]	Probability Est	EL	EEL
Brain tumor	AUC	0.687	0.963	0.974	**0.976**
	F-score	0.551	0.428	0.482	**0.592**
Cochlea	AUC	0.687	0.963	0.974	**0.976**
	F-score	0.223	0.239	0.431	**0.631**
Surgical instr.	AUC	0.346	0.949	0.959	**0.985**
	F-score	0.239	0.711	0.725	**0.851**
Optic disc	AUC	0.687	0.963	0.974	**0.976**
	F-score	0.506	0.367	0.494	**0.665**

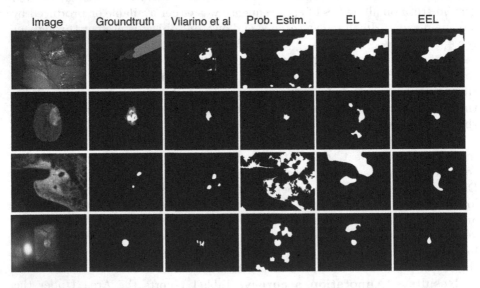

Fig. 4. Qualitative results. Each row shows a different dataset with an example image, the associated desired ground truth and the produced outcome of [9], using the probability estimation approach, EL approach and the proposed EEL. Binary images were generated by thresholding results at a 5% False Positive Rate.

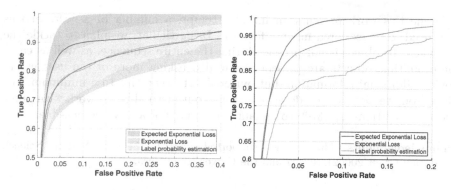

Fig. 5. (left) ROC performance variability on the same data but induced with different gaze sequences. (right) Performance in a crowd-sourcing setting.

Results – Gaze variance: In order to estimate the variance in annotations obtained with our strategy, 7 gaze observations were performed on the same laparoscopic image sequence. From these gaze observations, we ran our method on each set independently. Figure 5(left) shows the average ROC curve and standard error associated with our approach. In addition, we show similar performances when using the EL and when using the estimated labels only. On average we see that the EL does no better than the label estimation process, while the label estimation approach has slightly less variability. Overall, the EEL approach not only outperforms the other settings, but has lower variance as well.

Results – Crowd-Sourcing context: From the 7 gaze observations collected, we consider a Crowd-Sourcing context where the label estimation is combined as described in Sect. 4 in order to generate the associated ground truth. Figure 5(right) illustrates the performance attained when doing so. While the overall trend is no different to the previous experiment, the performance reached by the EEL approach is vastly higher. This is unsurprising given that more gaze information is provided in this setting (*i.e.* 7 annotators) and that more of the object is in fact viewed, yielding thus more positive samples, as well as better ϵ_S estimates.

6 Conclusion

In this work we have presented a strategy for domain experts to provide useful pixel-wise annotations in a passive way. By leveraging cheap eye gaze tracking technology, we have showed that gaze information can be used to produce segmentation ground truth in a variety of 3D or video imaging modalities. We achieved this by introducing a novel EEL function that is robust to large amounts of unlabeled data and few positive samples. We also demonstrated that our approach could be used in the context of crowd-sourcing where multiple annotators are available.

While this work presents an initial attempt, a number of aspects of this work need to be explored moving forward. In particular, we plan to tackle the case when the object is not present during the entire sequence, as well as cases where multiple objects are present. Naturally, asking more of the user would provide additional information, but our goal is to keep this to a minimum. For this reason, we also plan on determining how our method could work with noisy object observations, as %100 compliant users may not always be possible.

Acknowledgements. This work was supported in part by the Swiss National Science Foundation Grant 200021-162347 and the University of Bern.

References

1. Kamnitsas, K., Ledig, C., Newcombe, V., Simpson, J., Kane, A., Menon, D., Rueckert, D., Glocker, B.: Efficient multi-scale 3d cnn with fully connected crf for accurate brain lesion segmentation. Med. Image Anal. **36**, 61–78 (2017)
2. Anthimopoulos, M., Christodoulidis, S., Ebner, L., Christe, A., Mougiakakou, S.G.: Lung pattern classification for interstitial lung diseases using a deep convolutional neural network. IEEE Trans. Med. Imaging **35**(5), 1207–1216 (2016)
3. Konyushkova, K., Sznitman, R., Fua, P.: Introducing geometry in active learning for image segmentation. In: IEEE International Conference on Computer Vision (ICCV), pp. 2974–2982 (2015)
4. Mosinska-Domanska, A., Sznitman, R., Glowacki, P., Fua, P.: Active learning for delineation of curvilinear structures. In: IEEE Conference on Computer Vision and Pattern Recognition (CVPR), pp. 5231–5239 (2016)
5. Shin, H., Roth, H., Gao, M., Lu, L., Xu, Z., Nogues, I., Yao, J., Mollura, D., Summers, R.: Deep convolutional neural networks for computer-aided detection: Cnn architectures, dataset characteristics and transfer learning. IEEE Trans. Med. Imaging **35**(5), 1285–1298 (2016)
6. Bermúdez-Chacón, R., Becker, C., Salzmann, M., Fua, P.: Scalable unsupervised domain adaptation for electron microscopy. In: Ourselin, S., Joskowicz, L., Sabuncu, M.R., Unal, G., Wells, W. (eds.) MICCAI 2016. LNCS, vol. 9901, pp. 326–334. Springer, Cham (2016). doi:10.1007/978-3-319-46723-8_38
7. Maier-Hein, L., et al.: Can masses of non-experts train highly accurate image classifiers? In: Golland, P., Hata, N., Barillot, C., Hornegger, J., Howe, R. (eds.) MICCAI 2014. LNCS, vol. 8674, pp. 438–445. Springer, Cham (2014). doi:10.1007/978-3-319-10470-6_55
8. Cheplygina, V., Perez-Rovira, A., Kuo, W., Tiddens, H.A.W.M., de Bruijne, M.: Early experiences with crowdsourcing airway annotations in chest CT. In: Carneiro, G., et al. (eds.) LABELS/DLMIA -2016. LNCS, vol. 10008, pp. 209–218. Springer, Cham (2016). doi:10.1007/978-3-319-46976-8_22
9. Vilariño, F., Lacey, G., Zhou, J., Mulcahy, H., Patchett, S.: Automatic labeling of colonoscopy video for cancer detection. In: Iberian Conference on Pattern Recognition and Image Analysis, pp. 290–297 (2007)
10. Sadeghi, M., Tien, G., Hamarneh, G., Atkins, M.S.: Hands-free interactive image segmentation using eyegaze. In: Proceedings SPIE, Medical Imaging Computer-Aided Diagnosis, p. 7260 (2009)

11. Khosravan, N., Celik, H., Turkbey, B., Cheng, R., McCreedy, E., McAuliffe, M., Bednarova, S., Jones, E., Chen, X., Choyke, P., Wood, P., Bagci, U.: Gaze2segment: a pilot study for integrating eye-tracking technology into medical image segmentation. In: MICCAI, Workshop on Medical Computer Vision: Algorithms for Big Data (2016)
12. Chang, J., Wei, D., Fisher III., J.W.: A video representation using temporal superpixels. In: IEEE Conference on Computer Vision and Pattern Recognition (CVPR), pp. 2051–2058 (2013)
13. Hastie, T., Tibshirani, R., Friedman, J.: Data mining, inference, and prediction. The Elements of Statistical Learning. SSS. Springer, New York (2009)
14. Sermanet, P., Eigen, D., Zhang, X., Mathieu, M., Fergus, R., Lecun, Y.: Overfeat: integrated recognition, localization and detection using convolutional networks. In: International Conference on Learning Representations (2014)
15. Zhou, D., Bousquet, O., Lal, T., Weston, J., Schölkopf, B.: Learning with local and global consistency. In: Advances in Neural Information Processing Systems, pp. 321–328 (2003)
16. Menze, B.E.: The multimodal brain tumor image segmentation benchmark (BRATS). IEEE Trans. Med. Imaging 34(10), 1993–2024 (2014)

SwifTree: Interactive Extraction of 3D Trees Supporting Gaming and Crowdsourcing

Mian Huang[✉] and Ghassan Hamarneh

Medical Image Analysis Lab, School of Computing Science,
Simon Fraser University, Burnaby, BC, Canada
{mianh,hamarneh}@sfu.ca

Abstract. Analysis of vascular and airway trees of circulatory and respiratory systems is important for many clinical applications. Automatic segmentation of these tree-like structures from 3D data remains an open problem due to their complex branching patterns, geometrical diversity, and pathology. On the other hand, it is challenging to design intuitive interactive methods that are practical to use in 3D for trees with tens or hundreds of branches. We propose SwifTree, an interactive software for tree extraction that supports crowdsourcing and gamification. Our experiments demonstrate that: (i) aggregating the results of multiple SwifTree crowdsourced sessions achieves more accurate segmentation; (ii) using the proposed game-mode reduces time needed to achieve a pre-set tree segmentation accuracy; and (iii) SwifTree outperforms automatic segmentation methods especially with respect to noise robustness.

1 Introduction

Analysis of anatomical branching trees in the human body (i.e. vascular and airway trees of circulatory and respiratory systems) is important for a wide range of application (e.g., [22,24]). There are numerous methods for segmenting tree-like structures from 2D and 3D images, which may be generally classified into automatic (e.g., [5,15]) and interactive (e.g., [2,8,12,20,21,26]). Fully automatic tree segmentation methods are not yet completely accurate and reliable as they are often sensitive to parameters setting, are prone to leaking into nearby structures or to missing true bifurcating branches [15]. On the other hand, among interactive methods, optimal path techniques are commonly employed, which require the definition of start and end points (seeds) for each target branch (e.g., vessel) [8,26]. Other works proposed manual correction techniques to be applied after automatic segmentation [20,27]. Generally, interactive methods are hard to design and utilizing them for complex branching 3D trees with tens or hundreds of branches, which is not uncommon, is impractical.

There is a growing need for large numbers of segmented 3D imaging datasets for training machine learning systems and for validating newly proposed methods, however, there is a scarcity of segmented complex 3D trees. This work, which leverages gamification and crowdsourcing, is a first step towards enabling the collection of large numbers of segmented anatomical trees.

© Springer International Publishing AG 2017
M.J. Cardoso et al. (Eds.): CVII-STENT/LABELS 2017, LNCS 10552, pp. 116–125, 2017.
DOI: 10.1007/978-3-319-67534-3_13

The objective of gamification is to transform a mundane task into an immersive and engaging experience. Gamification has been leveraged in many ways, e.g., improving work productivity, patient rehabilitation, education and enhancing cognitive skills, etc. Crowdsourcing, on the other hand, provides a possible source of labelled (so called ground truth) data by leveraging humans' cognitive abilities and intelligence. Crowdsourcing is increasing in popularity and target applications, e.g., missing person search, disaster management, astronomy, and rehabilitation.

Table 1. Comparison of closest works. The meanings of the column headings are as follows. Crowd: method leverages crowdsourcing; Game: offers a "game" mode; MIA: designed for medical image analysis; 3D: handles 3D data; View: provides a view within the 3D volume; Control: controls the viewing position and angle; Tree: supports extracting branching tree-like structures; Skeleton: extracts centerline; Hierarchy: generates abstract representation of tree hierarchy.

Work	Crowd	Game	MIA	3D	View	Control	Tree	Skeleton	Hierarchy
Donath et al. [9]	✓								
Albarqouni et al. [3]	✓		✓						
Maier-Hein et al. [19]	✓		✓						
Chavez-Aragon et al. [6]	✓		✓						
Maier et al. [18]	✓		✓						
Luengo et al. [17]	✓	✓	✓						
Albarqouni et al. [4]	✓	✓	✓						
Hennersperger et al. [13]	✓	✓	✓						
Sommer et al. [23]			✓	✓			✓		
Poon et al. [21]			✓				✓	✓	
Vickerman et al. [26]			✓				✓	✓	✓
Abeysinghe et al. [2]			✓	✓			✓	✓	
Yu et al. [27]			✓	✓			✓	✓	✓
Marks et al. [20]			✓	✓			✓	✓	✓
Straka et al. [25]			✓	✓	✓		✓		
Abdoulaev et al. [1]			✓	✓	✓		✓		
Edmond et al. [10]			✓	✓	✓		✓	✓	
Coburn et al. [7]	✓	✓	✓	✓	✓	✓			
Heng et al. [12]			✓	✓	✓		✓	✓	✓
Diepenbrock et al. [8]			✓	✓	✓		✓	✓	✓
Proposed SwifTree	✓	✓	✓	✓	✓	✓	✓	✓	✓

Table 1 contrasts our proposed work with some of the most related literature. Although there has been several works that deployed gamification and/or crowdsourcing for medical image analysis, to the best of our knowledge, this is the first work to utilize gamification and crowdsourcing for vascular/airway tree extraction from 3D images. We argue that without the user confirming the segmentation everywhere along all branches of the tree, there is significant possibility of erroneously segmented regions. Therefore, we set out to develop SwifTree, a tool that allows the user to quickly and intuitively traverse and extract the anatomical tree in its entirety in a 3D volume, while supporting and leveraging gamification and crowdsourcing. Briefly, using SwifTree, the operator steers their way down along the bifurcating tree branches using intuitive controls. To address the mundane and time-consuming nature of delineating many branches, SwifTree employ gamification concepts. Finally, leveraging crowdsourcing, SwifTree allows multiple users to cooperate and generate multiple results that are then aggregated to produce the final extracted tree.

2   Method

Overview: After a 3D image is loaded into SwifTree, the image is processed to extract image features for controlling the properties of glyphs placed in a 3D scene to provide helpful cues to the user. In order to provide the user with multiple alternative views of the 3D scene, multiple virtual cameras at suitable vantage points are used. Each user is provided with controls (e.g. keyboard shortcuts) to facilitate navigating through the tree within the 3D image. In the crowdsourcing setup, the users travel virtually through the tree branches to construct trees in, both, a 3D spatial layout and in an abstract graph tree representation (an example is shown in Fig. 1). The results are aggregated to yield the final extracted tree and graph. The details follow.

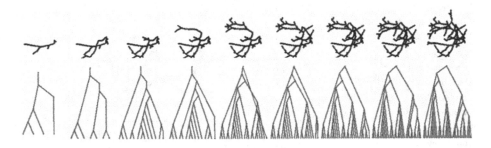

Fig. 1. Illustration of the sequence of steps which SwifTree uses to extract a 3D tree. Top: 3D spatial domain; bottom: corresponding abstract tree graph.

Image processing and glyph visualization: Figure 2 shows a schematic of the components that comprise a SwifTree 3D scene. The user interrogates different locations within the volume via a 3D polyhedral cursor. In a first attempt to visualize the image data for the user, we found that surface rendering (via marching cubes) and volume rendering (e.g. via ray casting) of the image data to overcrowd the scene. Instead we used slices and glyphs as described next. A grayscale oblique slice, cutting through the 3D volume, is rendered facing the user's viewing direction so that the slice would depict the cross-section of a branch as a single bright disk. As the user moves towards a bifurcation, the disk gradually splits into two, one for each child branch. We also render gradient glyphs based on the 3D image intensity gradient to highlight an estimate of the surface boundary surrounding the tree branches. To highlight the voxels in the interior to tree branches, we use tree-core glyphs calculated using the Frangi filter [11]. We experimented with different glyph densities (i.e. at every voxel or not), opacity values, sizes and shapes, and found the following settings to provide useful cues with minimal clutter: the size of each glyph was close to the size of a single voxel; the glyphs were rendered only at voxels with a strong response (i.e. gradient magnitude and tubularness surpassed an empirically-set threshold); and the opacity of a glyph was set proportional to the response magnitude. 3D glyphs were used for the tree-core glyphs but, for the gradient glyphs, flat 2D polygons with their normals pointing along the gradient direction were used in order to visually capture the local edges. Additionally, two virtual cameras are added to the scene: one camera provides a first-person local view whereas the other displays a more global bird's-eye view.

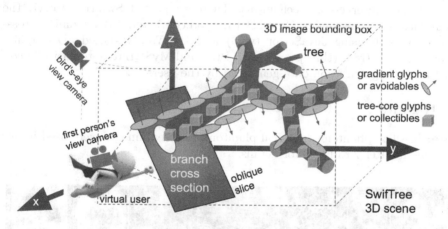

Fig. 2. Elements of SwifTree 3D scene (see text).

Navigation and movement: The aforementioned 3D cursor can be moved and rotated interactively by the user (move-forward, rotate-left, etc.). Additionally, once the user encounters a bifurcation (by observing the branch cross-section splitting), they press a key to *push* the current state parameters (i.e. location and camera viewpoints) into a *bifurcation stack*. After the user traverses one of the child branches (and optionally the grandchild branches), they *pop* the state parameters, to move the cursor and cameras back up the tree hierarchy to a previously-identified bifurcation location, so that the other child branches can be explored. Note that a trail of glyphs is left along the path explored by the user in order to ensure that the user does not explore the same branch twice.

Interactive and game mode: In SwifTree's game-mode, the cursor is an avatar that possesses a velocity controlled by the player. The player navigates the 3D volume by 'flying' through branches and identifying bifurcation locations using game-like controls (e.g., speed up, slow down, turn left). Also in game mode, the tree-core glyphs are set to be *collectibles*, i.e., as the user's cursor passes over these glyphs, they are collected and hidden with an accompanying sound effect and a score increment. The gradient glyphs, on the other hand, are *avoidables* that reduce the score, since they represent branch boundaries that should not be crossed. In SwifTree's non-game interactive mode, the user's cursor can be seen as an inertia-less paintbrush manipulated by the user.

Crowdsourcing and aggregation: We recruit multiple users or players to carry out a tree (or part of the tree) extraction session. The collected tree branches for the same image across all sessions are first unioned together and then a 3D spherical kernel is used to perform morphological closing. Then a medial axis transform is applied to extract the tree skeleton and network analysis is performed to create the abstract graph tree representation [14].

Implementation details: We used MATLAB (R2015b) to test several visualization and interaction mechanisms. Then we ported SwifTree to: (i) the cross-platform game engine Unity3D (unity3d.com) and (ii) an online cross-browser version using JavaScript (v6.0) and the WebGL-based 3D graphics library Three.js (r83) (threejs.org), with PHP and MySQL to automatically collect the tree segmentation data generated by the users.

3 Results

Data: In-silico phantoms, physical phantom, and real images were used in our experiments. Refer to Fig. 3 for details.

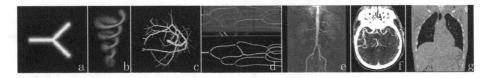

Fig. 3. Datasets: (a–c) In-silico phantoms: Y-Junc ($60 \times 60 \times 60$ voxels; 1 mm isotropic voxel), Helix ($50 \times 50 \times 100$; 1 mm isotropic), and VascuSynth ($101 \times 101 \times 101$; 1 mm isotropic); (d) Physical phantom ($168 \times 168 \times 159$; 1 mm isotropic); (e) Renal MRA ($576 \times 448 \times 72$; $0.625 \times 0.625 \times 1.4\,\mathrm{mm}^3$); (f) Brain CTA ($352 \times 448 \times 176$; $0.5134 \times 0.5134 \times 0.8\,\mathrm{mm}^3$); (g) Airways in CT ($512 \times 512 \times 587$; $0.5859 \times 0.5859 \times 0.6\,\mathrm{mm}^3$).

Supplementary material: The reader is referred to a simplified web-based version of SwifTree at http://swiftree-org.stackstaging.com and to the supplementary video https://youtu.be/AReIFQc47H4.

Evaluation criteria: We adopt the following criteria as described by Lo et al. [16]: branch count (BC); branches detected (BD); tree length (TL); tree length detected (TLD); leakage count (LC); and false positive rate (FPR).

Table 2. Accuracy of tree extraction by ITK-Snap, Gorgon and SwifTree. Highest accuracy in bold.

Data	Y-Junc			Helix			VascuSynth			Phantom			Kidney			Brain			Airway		
Tool	ITK-Snap	Gorgon	SwifTree	ITK-Snap	Gorgon	SwifTree	ITK-Snap	Gorgon	SwifTree	ITK-Snap	Gorgon	SwifTree	ITK-Snap	Gorgon	SwifTree	ITK-Snap	Gorgon	SwifTree	ITK-Snap	Gorgon	SwifTree
BC	3	1	**3**	**3**	1	**3**	58	27	**87**	47	28	**52**	13	5	**21**	30	†	**82**	57	†	**151**
BD(%)	**100**	33	**100**	**100**	33	**100**	52	24	**79**	72	43	**80**	56	21	**91**	24	†	**65**	19	†	**51**
TL(cm)	4	1	**5**	15	1	**22**	75	40	**99**	90	56	84	40	19	**47**	34	†	**64**	28	†	**91**
TLD(%)	86	5	**90**	51	1	**75**	53	28	**70**	**77**	48	72	55	27	**66**	30	†	**56**	17	†	**55**
LC	1	2	**1**	35	1	**5**	273	**85**	152	45	98	**27**	57	9	**1**	82	†	144	81	†	284
FPR(%)	2	85	**1**	37	97	**1**	59	72	**14**	9	43	**4**	42	79	**5**	19	†	**12**	**11**	†	19

†: software froze and could not handle the complex tree.

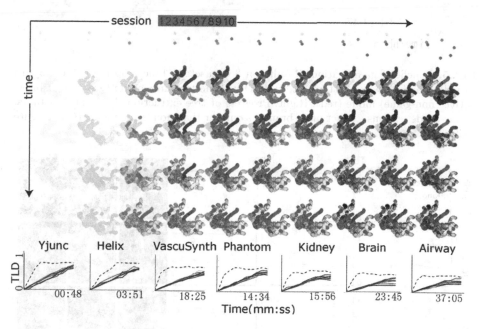

Fig. 4. Benefits of crowdsourcing. Top: The temporal progress of each of 10 sessions running SwifTree on the Brain dataset. As time advances and more sessions are included, the aggregated tree becomes more accurate and complete. Bottom: Plots of TLD vs time, for all data sets. Each solid colored curve corresponds to one tree extraction session. The black dashed curve, with better tree detection (i.e. higher than other curves), corresponds to the aggregated tree from all 10 sessions.

Tree extraction accuracy: Table 2 compares SwifTree to the ITK-Snap (itksnap.org) and Gorgon (gorgon.wustl.edu) tools. In ITK-Snap the user had to visit different slices to annotate pixels as tree branches, whereas in Gorgon, the user selected the end points of branches. We see that SwifTree gives the highest BD accuracy for all datasets, the highest TLD for all datasets except Phantom, and the lowest FPR for all datasets except Airway.

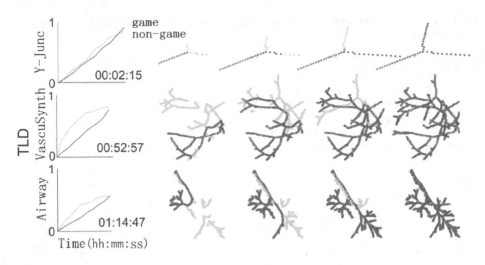

Fig. 5. Benefit of gamification. Results on 3 dataset: Y-Junc (top row); VascuSynth (middle); and Airway (bottom). Left: TLD vs time for game-mode (green) and interactive (non-game) mode (red). Right: Progress of tree extraction shown at 4 instants. Game-mode sessions extract more branches quicker than non-game mode. (Color figure online)

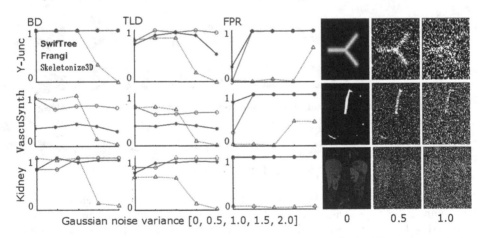

Fig. 6. Robustness to noise. Left: Comparison of Frangi filter, ImageJ Skeletonize3D and SwifTree in terms of robustness to noise. BD, TLD, and FPR are reported for the 3 methods across 3 datasets: Y-Junc (top), VascuSynth (middle) and Kidney (bottom). Right: Sample slices from each dataset at selected noise levels for illustration.

Benefit of crowdsourcing: We collected the results from 10 tree extraction sessions for each dataset using SwifTree (i.e., 70 sessions). The results are aggregated to obtain a single tree per dataset. As can be seen in Fig. 5, the tree aggregated from all participating sessions gives a more complete tree than any of the trees from the individual sessions. Also, the aggregated tree has the highest tree length detected with the highest initial slope (i.e. fastest increase). A small dip can be seen in the TLD of the aggregated tree due to false positive branches from some sessions.

Benefit of gamification: Figure 4 shows that enabling SwifTree game-mode features (i.e. velocity, sound effects, score, collectibles, and avoidables) reduces the time needed to reconstruct a pre-set tree compared to the non-game mode.

Robustness to noise: In Fig. 6, we compare SwifTree's results to those obtained by Frangi filter and ImageJ Skeletonize3D plug-in under different levels of Gaussian noise. We see that Frangi filter and Skeletonize3D report high detection rates of branches and trees (top and middle rows). However, they suffer from a high number of false positives (bottom row). SwifTree's false positive rate is much lower.

4   Conclusion

We proposed SwifTree, a novel tool for extracting tree-like structures from 3D images. We showed that by leveraging gamification and crowdsourcing, SwifTree can achieve more accurate results faster and is more robust to noise than traditional segmentation tools. The next phase of our work involves releasing SwifTree publicly as a "Human Intelligence Task" (HIT) on the established crowdsourcing platform Amazon Mechanical Turk, then analyzing the results collected from a large scale study involving hundreds of workers or "Turkers". There are several directions to explore that can improve the performance of the tool, such as more elaborate game design (e.g. improved visualization, sound, scoring system, and game-levels); an aggregation approach that gives higher weights to more expert users; detecting branch thickness; as well as performing large-scale user studies.

References

1. Abdoulaev, G., Cadeddu, S., Delussu, G., Donizelli, M., Formaggia, L., Giachetti, A., Gobbetti, E., Leone, A., Manzi, C., Pili, P., et al.: ViVa: the virtual vascular project. IEEE Trans. Inform. Technol. Biomed. **2**(4), 268–274 (1998)
2. Abeysinghe, S.S., Ju, T.: Interactive skeletonization of intensity volumes. Vis. Comput. **25**(5–7), 627–635 (2009)
3. Albarqouni, S., Baur, C., Achilles, F., Belagiannis, V., Demirci, S., Navab, N.: Aggnet: deep learning from crowds for mitosis detection in breast cancer histology images. IEEE Trans. Med. Imaging **35**(5), 1313–1321 (2016)
4. Albarqouni, S., Matl, S., Baust, M., Navab, N., Demirci, S.: Playsourcing: a novel concept for knowledge creation in biomedical research. In: Carneiro, G., et al. (eds.) LABELS/DLMIA -2016. LNCS, vol. 10008, pp. 269–277. Springer, Cham (2016). doi:10.1007/978-3-319-46976-8_28
5. Cetin, S., Demir, A., Yezzi, A., Degertekin, M., Unal, G.: Vessel tractography using an intensity based tensor model with branch detection. TMI **32**(2), 348–363 (2013)
6. Chávez-Aragón, A., Lee, W.-S., Vyas, A.: A crowdsourcing web platform-hip joint segmentation by non-expert contributors. In: MeMeA, pp. 350–354. IEEE (2013)

7. Coburn, C.: Play to cure: genes in space. Lancet Oncol. **15**(7), 688 (2014)
8. Diepenbrock, S., Ropinski, T.: From imprecise user input to precise vessel segmentations. In: VCBM. EG, pp. 65–72 (2012)
9. Donath, A., Kondermann, D.: Is crowdsourcing for optical flow ground truth generation feasible? In: Chen, M., Leibe, B., Neumann, B. (eds.) ICVS 2013. LNCS, vol. 7963, pp. 193–202. Springer, Heidelberg (2013). doi:10.1007/978-3-642-39402-7_20
10. Edmond, E.C., Sim, S.X.-L., Li, H.-H., Tan, E.-K., Chan, L.-L.: Vascular tortuosity in relationship with hypertension and posterior fossa volume in hemifacial spasm. BMC Neurol. **16**, 120 (2016)
11. Frangi, A.F., Niessen, W.J., Vincken, K.L., Viergever, M.A.: Multiscale vessel enhancement filtering. In: Wells, W.M., Colchester, A., Delp, S. (eds.) MICCAI 1998. LNCS, vol. 1496, pp. 130–137. Springer, Heidelberg (1998). doi:10.1007/BFb0056195
12. Heng, P.-A., Sun, H., Chen, K.-W., Wong, T.-T.: Interactive navigation of virtual vessel tracking with 3D intelligent scissors. IJIG **1**(02), 273–285 (2001)
13. Hennersperger, C., Baust, M.: Play for me: image segmentation via seamless playsourcing. Comput. Games J. **6**(1–2), 1–16 (2017)
14. Kerschnitzki, M., Kollmannsberger, P., Burghammer, M., Duda, G.N., Weinkamer, R., Wagermaier, W., Fratzl, P.: Architecture of the osteocyte network correlates with bone material quality. JBMR **28**(8), 1837–1845 (2013)
15. Lesage, D., Angelini, E.D., Bloch, I., Funka-Lea, G.: A review of 3D vessel lumen segmentation techniques: models, features and extraction schemes. MIA **13**(6), 819–845 (2009)
16. Lo, P., Van Ginneken, B., JosephMReinhardt, T.Y., De Jong, P.A., Irving, B., Fetita, C., Ortner, M., Pinho, R., Sijbers, J., et al.: Extraction of airways from CT (EXACT'09). TMI **31**(11), 2093–2107 (2012)
17. Arranz, A., Frean, J.: Crowdsourcing malaria parasite quantification: an online game for analyzing images of infected thick blood smears. J. Med. Internet Res. **14**(6), e167 (2012)
18. Maier-Hein, L., et al.: Can masses of non-experts train highly accurate image classifiers? In: Golland, P., Hata, N., Barillot, C., Hornegger, J., Howe, R. (eds.) MICCAI 2014. LNCS, vol. 8674, pp. 438–445. Springer, Cham (2014). doi:10.1007/978-3-319-10470-6_55
19. Maier-Hein, L., et al.: Crowdsourcing for reference correspondence generation in endoscopic images. In: Golland, P., Hata, N., Barillot, C., Hornegger, J., Howe, R. (eds.) MICCAI 2014. LNCS, vol. 8674, pp. 349–356. Springer, Cham (2014). doi:10.1007/978-3-319-10470-6_44
20. Marks, P.C., Preda, M., Henderson, T., Liaw, L., Lindner, V., Friesel, R.E., Pinz, I.M.: Interactive 3D analysis of blood vessel trees and collateral vessel volumes in magnetic resonance angiograms in the mouse ischemic hindlimb model. OJMI **7**, 19 (2013)
21. Poon, K., Hamarneh, G., Abugharbieh, R.: Live-vessel: extending livewire for simultaneous extraction of optimal medial and boundary paths in vascular images. In: Ayache, N., Ourselin, S., Maeder, A. (eds.) MICCAI 2007. LNCS, vol. 4792, pp. 444–451. Springer, Heidelberg (2007). doi:10.1007/978-3-540-75759-7_54
22. Sankaran, S., Grady, L., Taylor, C.A.: Fast computation of hemodynamic sensitivity to lumen segmentation uncertainty. TMI **34**(12), 2562–2571 (2015)
23. Sommer, C., Straehle, C., Koethe, U., Hamprecht, F.A.: Ilastik: Interactive learning and segmentation toolkit. In: ISBI, pp. 230–233. IEEE (2011)

24. Sotelo, J., Urbina, J., Valverde, I., Tejos, C., Irarráazaval, P., Andia, M.E., Uribe, S., Hurtado, D.E.: 3D quantification of wall shear stress and oscillatory shear index using a finite-element method in 3D CINE PC-MRI data of the thoracic aorta. TMI **35**(6), 1475–1487 (2016)
25. Straka, M., Cervenansky, M., La Cruz, A., Kochl, A., Sramek, M., Groller, E., Fleischmann, D.: Focus & context visualization in CT-angiography. The Vessel-Glyph. IEEE (2004)
26. Vickerman, M.B., Keith, P.A., McKay, T.L., Gedeon, D.J., MichikoWatanabe, M.M., Karunamuni, G., Kaiser, P.K., Sears, J.E., Ebrahem, Q., et al.: VESGEN 2D: automated, user-interactive software for quantification and mapping of angiogenic and lymphangiogenic trees and networks. Anat. Rec. **292**(3), 320–332 (2009)
27. Yu, K.-C., Ritman, E.L., Higgins, W.E.: Graphical tools for improved definition of 3D arterial trees. In: Medical Imaging 2004. SPIE, pp. 485–495 (2004)

Crowdsourced Emphysema Assessment

Silas Nyboe Ørting[1(✉)], Veronika Cheplygina[2,5], Jens Petersen[1],
Laura H. Thomsen[3], Mathilde M.W. Wille[4], and Marleen de Bruijne[1,5]

[1] Department of Computer Science, University of Copenhagen,
Copenhagen, Denmark
silas@di.ku.dk
[2] Medical Image Analysis (IMAG/e), Department of Biomedical Engineering,
Eindhoven University of Technology, Eindhoven, The Netherlands
[3] Department of Respiratory Medicine, Gentofte Hospital, Hellerup, Denmark
[4] Department of Diagnostic Imaging, Bispebjerg Hospital, Copenhagen, Denmark
[5] Biomedical Imaging Group Rotterdam, Departments of Radiology and Medical
Informatics, Erasmus MC - University Medical Center Rotterdam,
Rotterdam, The Netherlands

Abstract. Classification of emphysema patterns is believed to be useful
for improved diagnosis and prognosis of chronic obstructive pulmonary
disease. Emphysema patterns can be assessed visually on lung CT scans.
Visual assessment is a complex and time-consuming task performed by
experts, making it unsuitable for obtaining large amounts of labeled data.
We investigate if visual assessment of emphysema can be framed as an
image similarity task that does not require expert. Substituting untrained
annotators for experts makes it possible to label data sets much faster
and at a lower cost. We use crowd annotators to gather similarity triplets
and use t-distributed stochastic triplet embedding to learn an embedding.
The quality of the embedding is evaluated by predicting expert assessed
emphysema patterns. We find that although performance varies due to
low quality triplets and randomness in the embedding, we still achieve a
median F_1 score of 0.58 for prediction of four patterns.

Keywords: Crowdsourcing · Emphysema · Similarity learning

1 Introduction

Emphysema is a lung pathology common to chronic obstructive pulmonary disease that is a major cause of morbidity and mortality world wide [3]. Emphysema
is characterized by destruction of lung tissue. Lung CT scans can reveal emphysema and visual scoring can be used to rate the extent and type of emphysema
in the lungs [14]. Visual scores can be used for training classifiers to automatically assess presence and extent of emphysema [9,11]. However, visual scoring of
emphysema by experts is both expensive and prone to high rater disagreement
[14]. Instead of performing a full visual scoring, which requires expert knowledge

© Springer International Publishing AG 2017
M.J. Cardoso et al. (Eds.): CVII-STENT/LABELS 2017, LNCS 10552, pp. 126–135, 2017.
DOI: 10.1007/978-3-319-67534-3_14

of the lungs, we investigate whether it is possible to reduce emphysema assessment to a simpler task that can be performed by untrained raters, or crowds.

In fields such as computer vision, crowdsourcing - outsourcing simple tasks to a crowd of online users, often without any specific training - has been used successfully to gather labels for training and validation of classifiers [4]. Most of this research focuses on collecting labels that directly characterize the content of the image, for instance presence of an object or indicating regions of interest. Motivated by the fact that some categorization tasks may be difficult for non-experts, a few others instead focus on collecting assessments of similarities between images. For example, Wah et al. [13] collect similarities between images of different bird species, which most people do not know by name, but can easily assess their visual similarity. The similarities can then be used to learn an embedding that can aid classification.

Due to the success of crowdsourcing in computer vision, there have also been several efforts to apply it to medical imaging [1,2,6,8]. Similar to methods from the computer vision field, these works focus on collecting labels for images, targeting classification or segmentation tasks. For example, the crowd can be asked to grade retinal images as normal or abnormal [8] or to segment airways in 2D slices of chest CT images [2]. To the best of our knowledge, this work is the first to gather crowdsourced similarities for medical images, as well as to apply a crowdsourcing approach to classification of emphysema patterns.

2 Materials and Methods

2.1 Data

We used 40 chest CT scans from the a national lung cancer screening trial [10] and visual assessment of emphysema from [14]. Visual assessment is performed by considering the full 3D volume and splitting each lung in three regions. The top, middle and lower regions are defined as above carina, between carina and inferior pulmonary vein, and below inferior pulmonary vein. The volume is assigned a label indicating the predominant emphysema pattern and each region is assigned an estimate of the extent of emphysema in the region. The 40 scans were selected amongst those where raters agreed on visual assessment of both predominant pattern and emphysema extent in the upper right region. We excluded scans with panlobular emphysema due to low prevalence. We grouped candidate scans based on predominant pattern: normal (N), centrilobular (C), paraseptal (P), mixed (M), and chose ten scans from each group. For the three emphysema groups (C, P, M) we chose the scans with highest extent, and for the normal group we chose ten scans at random. We used lung fields segmented from the scans obtained from [5].

We extracted nine coronal slices from the top region of the right lung of each scan. The slices were evenly spaced (10 mm) and located such that the center slice coincided with the center slice of the region. In this way we covered a depth of 80 mm and avoided slices at the very boundary of the lungs. An example of an extracted set of slices is given in Fig. 1. The slices are extracted from a subject with a large extent of centrilobular emphysema. We see that while texture patterns vary a lot throughout the region, patterns are similar between neighboring slices. It is also clear that size and shape of the lung region varies with slice location. To avoid having workers focus on the differences in lung size and shape, we stratify slices by their location in the lung when sampling triplets.

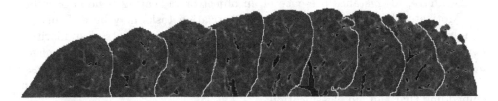

Fig. 1. Nine slices extracted from a single volume. There is a large extent of centrilobular emphysema. We can see that neighboring slices tend to have more similar texture patterns than slices that are far away from each other. White border added for clarity.

2.2 Crowdsourced Triplets

We used Amazon MTurk[1] to collect similarity triplets. MTurk centers on the concept of a human intelligence task (HIT), a self-contained task that can be solved by a worker. We designed our HIT as a set of three image triplets where the task is to provide similarity assessment of each of the three triplets. A screenshot showing part of a HIT is given in Fig. 2. We asked workers to choose one of two images on the right with the most similar disease patterns to the image on the left. We instructed workers to look for emphysema patterns, defined as areas of low intensity, and consider the distribution of patterns of these areas: scattered throughout the lung or concentrated. We emphasized that workers should ignore differences in size and shape of the lung. We asked three different workers to perform each HIT. We required workers that had at least 1000 previously approved HITs and a 95% approval rate. The reward for each task was $0.10.

We collected 9720 similarity triplets for 3240 unique image triplets. 150 different workers worked on the HITs, with a median number of HITs per worker of 6.5 (19.5 similarity triplets). The median work time per HIT was 55 s. The most productive worker submitted 131 HITs and the lowest work time for a HIT was 4 s. More than 92% of the HITs were finished within 30 min of the first HIT being available. The total cost was $388.80.

2.3 Similarity Embedding

We used t-distributed stochastic triplet embedding (t-STE) [12] to learn an n-dimensional Euclidean embedding from the similarity triplets. t-STE searches for an embedding X that maximizes the probability of observing the given triplets.

---

[1] https://www.mturk.com.

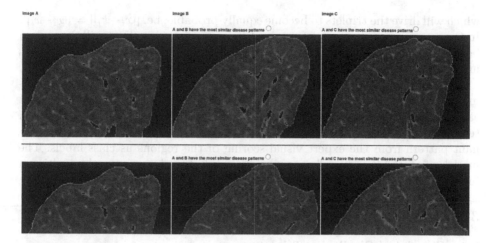

Fig. 2. Amazon MTurk user interface for collecting the similarity triplets

Let T be the set of known triplets and $ijl \in T$ a triplet indicating that $d(i,j) < d(i,l)$. The probability of ijl given $x_i, x_j, x_l \in X$ is

$$p_{ijl} = \frac{\left(1 + \frac{\|x_i - x_j\|_2}{\alpha}\right)^{-\frac{\alpha+1}{2}}}{\left(1 + \frac{\|x_i - x_j\|_2}{\alpha}\right)^{-\frac{\alpha+1}{2}} + \left(1 + \frac{\|x_i - x_l\|_2}{\alpha}\right)^{-\frac{\alpha+1}{2}}} \tag{1}$$

The optimization problem is

$$\min_X - \sum_{ijl \in T} \log p_{ijl} \tag{2}$$

which is solved with gradient descent using the implementation from Michael Wilber[2].

Crowdsourced similiarity triplets are very likely to contain inconsistent and redundant triplets. When multiple workers perform the same HIT this is definitely the case. McFee and Lanckriet [7] give empirical evidence that pruning triplets for consistency and redundancy reduces computation time without affecting performance. However, they compare against a baseline where directly disagreeing triplets are removed. Removing triplets where workers disagree removes information about the uncertainty of the triplets. We can implicitly model this uncertainty by keeping all triplets. It can be shown that for $x = x_i, x_j, x_l$ the conflicting triplets satisfy

$$\frac{\partial}{\partial x} p_{ijl} = -\frac{\partial}{\partial x} p_{ilj}, \tag{3}$$

and the sum of the derivatives becomes

$$\frac{\partial}{\partial x} \log p_{ijl} + \frac{\partial}{\partial x} \log p_{ilj} = \frac{\partial}{\partial x} p_{ijl} \left(\frac{1}{p_{ijl}} - \frac{1}{p_{ilj}}\right) \tag{4}$$

---

[2] https://github.com/gcr/cython_tste.

which will drive the triplets to become equally probable, i.e. $||x_i - x_j|| = ||x_i - x_l||$. In the case where ijl occur c_j times and ilj occur c_l the gradient will depend on both the ratio c_j/c_l and the distances $||x_i - x_j||, ||x_i - x_l||$. In this way workers uncertainty about triplets will be accounted for in the optimization.

We used k-fold cross-validation with a multinomial log-linear model to estimate the predictive performance of the obtained embeddings. We enforced that each test fold contained exactly one sample from each class. For four classes with ten scans each this resulted in 10-fold cross-validation. We used the predominant pattern from the expert visual scoring of the regions as class labels. The model was fitted as a neural network with one hidden layer using the multinom function from the nnet package[3].

3   Experiments and Results

3.1   Simulated Similarity Triplets

To estimate how many triplets are needed to reveal an underlying pattern we performed a simulation experiment. We defined a distance function that encodes a similarity hierarchy of visually assessed patterns and emphysema extent. Paraseptal emphysema often appear as a small number of large holes, whereas centrilobular emphysema often appear as a large number of small holes. We therefore expect most raters will consider normal and centrilobular patterns more similar than normal and paraseptal patterns. We also expect both centrilobular and paraseptal patterns to be considered more similar to the mixed pattern than to each other. For images with the same pattern class we used absolute distance on emphysema extent. This simple distance function does not account for variability in patterns and it is unlikely that image based similarity triplets will match the visual assessment perfectly. However, it does provide some insight into the amount of triplets necessary. We used three sets of randomly selected triplets with sizes of 120, 240, and 360. For each set of triplets we generated 100 2D embeddings and estimated the prediction performance of the embedding with the multinomial model described above. We used the F_1 score to measure performance

$$F_1 = 2 \cdot \frac{\text{precision} \cdot \text{recall}}{\text{precision} + \text{recall}}. \tag{5}$$

The median F_1 score for 120 triplets was 0.8 and improved to 0.9 for 240 triplets and to 1.0 for 360 triplets. There was some variation in performance for 120 and 240 triplets, whereas almost all 360 triplet embeddings gave perfect prediction. Representative embeddings for 120 and 240 triplets are given in Fig. 3. We can see that the embedding matches the distance function quite well, with normal and paraseptal being furthest from each other and mixed in between centrilobular and paraseptal. We also see some class overlap for 120 triplets and almost no overlap for 240 triplets. We used these results to guide the crowdsourcing to gather relatively many triplets for a small number of scans.

---

[3] https://cran.r-project.org/web/packages/nnet.

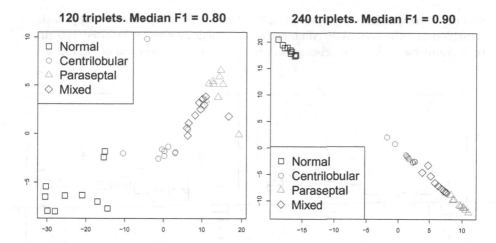

Fig. 3. Example embeddings from simulated triplets. Left: 120 triplets. Right: 240 triplets. While there is no overlap between emphysema and normal classes in both cases, there is some overlap between emphysema classes for 120 triplets.

3.2   Crowdsourced Similarity Triplets

We estimated the quality of the crowdsourced triplets by measuring the agreement with a small set of validation triplets. The validation triplets were labeled by one of the authors and consist of 52 triplets that the authors view as easy to reproduce. The overall agreement was 71% with a large variation between workers. We expected most workers to work on one or more validation triplets. However, due to the large number of workers only 41% of workers worked on a validation triplet and only 11% on more than two validation triplets. While agreement was lower than anticipated, and some workers had very poor agreement, we decided to include all triplets.

We varied the embedding dimensionality d from $1-10$. We set $\alpha = \max(d - 1, 1)$ for all experiments and used a random initialization of t-STE. From the similarity triplets we learned an embedding of slices. Due to the stratification of triplets by slice location it is not meaningful to embed different slice locations simultaneously. We therefore concatenated the slice feature vectors to obtain a region embedding. We normalized each slice embedding to avoid that slice locations with numerically large distances dominated the region embedding. As an alternative to embedding each slice location separately we added triplets between slice locations and embedded all slice locations simultaneously. The extra triplets were derived by exploiting that neighboring slices in a region, in general, are more similar than slices further away from each other. This "neighbor similarity" was encoded with the distance function

$$d(slice_i, slice_{i+1}) < d(slice_i, slice_{i+3}), \; i \in [1:6],$$
$$d(slice_i, slice_{i-1}) < d(slice_i, slice_{i-3}), \; i \in [4:9],$$

and the corresponding triplets were added to T. We refer to the first approach as stratified and the second as combined. All embeddings were repeated 100 times to account for variability arising from the random initialization of t-STE.

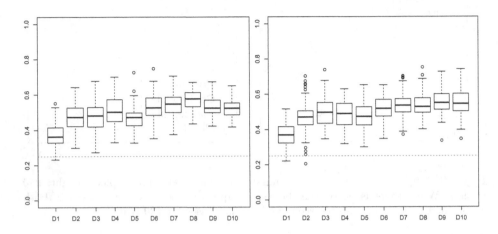

Fig. 4. Distribution of mean F_1 scores for classification of emphysema type. Left stratified, right combined. The dashed red line indicate random performance ($F_1 = 0.25$). (Color figure online)

Figure 4 shows the mean F_1 score over all classes for increasing embedding dimension for stratified and combined embeddings. Best median performance was achieved with D8 for stratified ($F_1 = 0.58$) and with D9 for combined ($F_1 = 0.55$). In both plots we see a large variation in performance. Adding the extra triplets for combined embedding seems to make performance more similar across dimensions, but does not decrease variation within each dimension. The direct source of the variation is the random initialization of t-STE. However, as the simulation showed, having a large consistent set of triplets will drive the variation in prediction performance to 0. The extra triplets for combined, that as subset is consistent, did not reduce variation, so the main underlying cause is likely having too many inconsistent triplets.

Figure 5 show performance by class. In all cases we see best performance on centrilobular and normal. For $D > 5$ we see consistently higher performance on centrilobular than on normal. Performance on centrilobular seems to be the main cause for the higher mean scores at D8 and D9. Treating mixed and paraseptal as one pattern makes the performance similar to performance on centrilobular (results not shown). This indicates that the main difficulty is in distinguishing paraseptal and mixed.

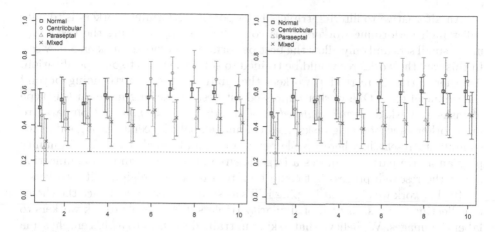

Fig. 5. F_1 scores for classification of emphysema type. Left for stratified, right for combined. The dashed red line indicate random performance ($F_1 = 0.25$). Symbols indicate median values and bars indicate ± 1 median absolute deviation. (Color figure online)

4   Discussion and Conclusion

Although there was large variation in prediction performance, it was in all but a few cases substantially better than random. The results from the simulation experiment show that more triplets improve median prediction performance and reduce variance. However, the simulation experiment uses triplets that perfectly encodes a distance function on patterns. While more crowdsourced triplets might improve performance and reduce variance, it is possible that higher quality set of triplets is needed to see significant gains.

Pruning triplets could improve quality. Directly inconsistent triplets, i.e. $ijl, ilj \in T$, can arise from poorly performing workers or difficult decisions. If we assume they represent difficult decisions, then they contain important information that we would like to keep. Pruning triplets is shown by [7] to be NP-hard and can only be solved approximately. Using the information from the direct inconsistencies to guide the pruning could be an interesting approach to improve the quality of the triplet set.

Direct inconsistencies due to poorly performing workers should not guide anything, but be removed. One approach is to rank workers and discard triplets from the least trustworthy workers. Ranking could be done by ensuring all workers perform tasks with a reference. Alternatively, it could be based on how well each worker agree with other workers. The first case requires expert labels and that each worker perform a minimum number of reference tasks. The second case requires that workers perform a large number of tasks and that tasks overlap with many different workers. In the future we intend to use one or both approaches to improve the quality of the triplet set.

An alternative to filtering triplets from poorly performing workers is to only enlist high performing workers. This could be done by splitting the tasks into many small sets and only allow the best performing workers to work on a new set. In this way the workforce would be trained to solve the tasks to our specification. Another option is recruiting workers that find the tasks worth doing beyond the financial gain. One worker expressed interest in working more on this type of tasks and asked *"Am I qualified to be a pulmonologist now?"*. Compared to many other crowdsourcing tasks, medical image analysis seems like a good fit for community research, where people outside the traditional research community play an active part. It requires a larger degree of openness and communication about the research process but could be a tool to recruit high quality workers.

In this work we aimed at keeping HITs as simple as possible, hence the choice of collecting triplets. Instead of similarity triplets it is possible to ask workers to label the images. We believe that asking untrained workers to assess emphysema pattern and extent would be overly optimistic. However, focusing on a few simple questions might work well, for example "Are there dark holes in the lung?", "Are holes present in more than a third of the lung?", "Are the holes predominantly at the boundary of the lung?". These types of questions correspond to a model we have of emphysema and could be used to derive emphysema pattern and extent labels. The downside is that we need to know exactly what we want answered at the risk of missing important unknowns in the data.

Regardless of the high variance in performance, we conclude that untrained crowd workers can perform emphysema assessment when it is framed as a question of image similarity. No quality assurance, beyond requiring that workers had experience with MTurk, was performed. It is likely that large improvements can be gained by quality assurance of similarity triplets.

Acknowledgments. We would like to thank family, friends and coworkers at the University of Copenhagen, Erasmus MC - University Medical Center Rotterdam, Eindhoven University of Technology, and the start-up understand.ai for their help in testing prototype versions of the crowdsourcing tasks. This study was financially supported by the Danish Council for Independent Research (DFF) and the Netherlands Organization for Scientific Research (NWO).

References

1. Albarqouni, S., Baur, C., Achilles, F., Belagiannis, V., Demirci, S., Navab, N.: Aggnet: deep learning from crowds for mitosis detection in breast cancer histology images. IEEE TMI **35**(5), 1313–1321 (2016)
2. Cheplygina, V., Perez-Rovira, A., Kuo, W., Tiddens, H.A.W.M., de Bruijne, M.: Early experiences with crowdsourcing airway annotations in chest CT. In: Carneiro, G., Mateus, D., Peter, L., Bradley, A., Tavares, J.M.R.S., Belagiannis, V., Papa, J.P., Nascimento, J.C., Loog, M., Lu, Z., Cardoso, J.S., Cornebise, J. (eds.) LABELS/DLMIA 2016. LNCS, vol. 10008, pp. 209–218. Springer, Cham (2016). doi:10.1007/978-3-319-46976-8_22
3. From the Global Strategy for the Diagnosis, Management and Prevention of COPD, Global Initiative for Chronic Obstructive Lung Disease (GOLD) (2015)

4. Kovashka, A., Russakovsky, O., Fei-Fei, L., Grauman, K.: Crowdsourcing in computer vision. Found. Trends. Comput. Graph. Vis. **10**(3), 177–243 (2016)
5. Lo, P., Sporring, J., Ashraf, H., Pedersen, J.J.H.: Vessel-guided airway tree segmentation: a voxel classification approach. Med. Image Anal. **14**(4), 527–538 (2010)
6. Maier-Hein, L., Mersmann, S., Kondermann, D., Bodenstedt, S., Sanchez, A., Stock, C., Kenngott, H.G., Eisenmann, M., Speidel, S.: Can masses of non-experts train highly accurate image classifiers? In: Golland, P., Hata, N., Barillot, C., Hornegger, J., Howe, R. (eds.) MICCAI 2014. LNCS, vol. 8674, pp. 438–445. Springer, Cham (2014). doi:10.1007/978-3-319-10470-6_55
7. McFee, B., Lanckriet, G.: Learning multi-modal similarity. J. Mach. Learn. Res. **12**, 491–523 (2011)
8. Mitry, D., Zutis, K., Dhillon, B., Peto, T., Hayat, S., Khaw, K.-T., Morgan, J.E., Moncur, W., Trucco, E., Foster, P.J.: The accuracy and reliability of crowdsource annotations of digital retinal images. Trans. Vis. Sci. Technol. **5**(5), 6–6 (2016)
9. Nishio, M., Nakane, K., Kubo, T., Yakami, M., Emoto, Y., Nishio, M., Togashi, K.: Automated prediction of emphysema visual score using homology-based quantification of low-attenuation lung region. PLOS ONE **12**(5), 1–12 (2017)
10. Pedersen, J.H., Ashraf, H., Dirksen, A., Bach, K., Hansen, H., Toennesen, P., Thorsen, H., Brodersen, J., Skov, B.G., Døssing, M., Mortensen, J., Richter, K., Clementsen, P., Seersholm, N.: The Danish randomized lung cancer CT screening trial-overall design and results of the prevalence round. J. Thorac. Oncol. **4**(5), 608–614 (2009)
11. Nyboe Ørting, S., Petersen, J., Wille, M., Thomsen, L., de Bruijne, M.: Quantifying emphysema extent from weakly labeled CT scans of the lungs using label proportions learning. In: MICCAI PIA, pp. 31–42. CreateSpace Independent Publishing Platform (2016)
12. van der Maaten, L., Weinberger, K.: Stochastic triplet embedding. In: IEEE MLSP, pp. 1–6 (2012)
13. Wah, C., Van Horn, G., Branson, S., Maji, S., Perona, P., Belongie, S.: Similarity comparisons for interactive fine-grained categorization. In: IEEE CVPR, pp. 859–866 (2014)
14. Wille, M.M., Thomsen, L.H., Dirksen, A., Petersen, J., Pedersen, J.H., Shaker, S.B.: Emphysema progression is visually detectable in low-dose CT in continuous but not in former smokers. Eur. Radiol. **24**(11), 2692–2699 (2014)

A Web-Based Platform for Distributed Annotation of Computerized Tomography Scans

Nicholas Heller[✉], Panagiotis Stanitsas, Vassilios Morellas,
and Nikolaos Papanikolopoulos

University of Minnesota Center for Distributed Robotics,
117 Pleasant St SE, Minneapolis, MN 55455, USA
{helle246,stani078,morellas,papan001}@umn.edu
http://distrob.cs.umn.edu

Abstract. Computer Aided Diagnosis (CAD) systems are adopting advancements at the forefront of computer vision and machine learning towards assisting medical experts with providing faster diagnoses. The success of CAD systems heavily relies on the availability of high-quality annotated data. Towards supporting the annotation process among teams of medical experts, we present a web-based platform developed for distributed annotation of medical images. We capitalize on the HTML5 canvas to allow for medical experts to quickly perform segmentation of regions of interest. Experimental evaluation of the proposed platform show a significant reduction in the time required to perform the annotation of abdominal computerized tomography images. Furthermore, we evaluate the relationship between the size of the harvested regions and the quality of the annotations. Finally, we present additional functionality of the developed platform for the closer examination of 3D point clouds for kidney cancer.

1 Introduction

Medical imaging modalities contain a wealth of useful information for the diagnosis of a wide range of ailments, rendering them an essential component of the diagnostic process. A plethora of tools for the accurate identification of risk markers for different pathologies in medical images has been developed (e.g. [2–6]). Such inference schemes require large amounts of annotated data, which are used for the training of supervised or semi-supervised models. Unfortunately, the very high cost of the annotation process associated with medical images results in a lack of publicly available benchmarks (e.g. [8,9]). The high cost can be attributed to the requirement of highly trained experts for providing the annotations. This scarcity of annotated data is prohibitive to the development of Computer Aided Diagnosis (CAD) for a variety of pathologies.

The overall objective of this study is concerned with the development of a CAD scheme for the localization and the health assessment of kidneys from abdominal Computerized Tomography (CT) scans. In that direction, two sub-problems can be identified; first the accurate localization and segmentation of

M.J. Cardoso et al. (Eds.): CVII-STENT/LABELS 2017, LNCS 10552, pp. 136–145, 2017.
DOI: 10.1007/978-3-319-67534-3_15

the organ (kidney) and the aorta and, second, the automated identification of abnormal masses (malignant tissue, benign tissue and cysts).

With the support of our medical collaborators, a collection of several hundred abdominal CT scans of kidney cancer patients has been acquired. A majority of the patients' pathologies are clear cell Renal Cell Carcinomas (RCCs) but papillary RCCs, angiomyolipomas, renal oncocytomas, and papillary urothelials are represented as well. Our intention is to create a rich collection of accurate delineations of abnormalities developed by the kidneys. This introduces an annotation burden which is distributed among urologists at different locations.

A large variety of tools is available for the generic annotation of images. Such tools were designed with much different tasks in mind and have a large number of extraneous features which, for an application like the one in hand, would unnecessarily increase the complexity of the annotation sessions. Two examples of such tools are the GNU Image Manipulation Program[1] and Adobe Photoshop[2].

Furthermore, the anticipated high data volume creates the need for a centralized storage and backup platform. In that way, users are not required to manually update annotation repositories after each session, and only necessitates redundancies at the server level, rather than the personal computer level.

2 Related Work

A number of specialized tools tailored to the task of high-volume image annotation have been created. One such platform is the Automated Slide Analysis Platform (ASAP)[3]. ASAP was built for the specific task of annotating whole slide histopathology images. It includes a large collection of tools for this task including the ability to draw polygons from sets of points and to create splines.

According to our partnering medical experts, certain features of ASAP are more relevant to the annotation of histopathological data. In our case, the most convenient way to segment our regions of interest was to simply draw outlines and fill them. Therefore, many of ASAP's features are vestigial to our task and would introduce unnecessary complexity. Additionally, ASAP is a desktop tool which requires the users to store a copy of the data locally. This is not ideal for our task for the reasons discussed in the previous section. Further, in order to save an annotation and move on to the next image or feature, at least 5 clicks are required by the user, on top of decisions he or she must make about where to store the annotation and which file to open next. This introduces a significant amount of unnecessary work which frustrates users and reduces efficiency.

Another platform that was created for this task is MIT CSAIL's LabelMe [1] website. This platform is well-made and better suited for our task than ASAP since it is web-based with central data management and requires only a single

---

[1] https://www.gimp.org/.
[2] https://www.adobe.com/products/photoshop.html.
[3] https://github.com/GeertLitjens/ASAP.

click to move to the next image. However, it is missing features which are critically important to our design objective. For instance, the tool only supports drawing using point-defined polygons. According to the experts we talked to, this is not ideal. Additionally, LabelMe draws with full opacity, and a simple experiment showed us that full opacity leads to higher variability among annotators and overall lower accuracies. Furthermore, the LabelMe interface does not have a "previous" button which medical experts told us was essential to their ability to accurately annotate, presumably so that they could conveniently flip back and forth between sequential frames in order to make better informed decisions about which regions are which.

In contrast, our platform was designed with the following three core requirements, namely, (i) distributed capabilities, (ii) robust and secure centralized data storage and, (iii) a lightweight interface focusing on the task in hand. Our use of the HTML5 canvas element makes this realizable. Additionally, in order to ensure a user-friendly presentation, our platform capitalizes on the Bootstrap[4] framework.

3   The Interface

The interface of the developed scheme was based on the the Bootstrap framework. In particular, we used Start Bootstrap's SB Admin template[5], since it allows for the *landing* page to provide the user with information on the state of the system. In our case, this is to display the annotation progress on a particular project. This landing page is depicted in Fig. 1. When the user clicks on the

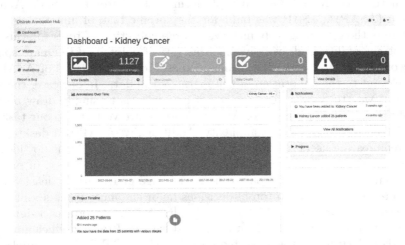

Fig. 1. The four colored cards correspond to the number of images belonging to each of the four bins: unannotated, pending, validated, and rejected. The proportions in each bin are visualized by the graph below the cards. This screen capture was taken when no images were yet annotated. (Color figure online)

---

[4] http://getbootstrap.com/.
[5] https://startbootstrap.com/template-overviews/sb-admin/.

unannotated card or the *annotate* button on the top left, it brings them to the image-set selection page. Here, the user sees a vertical list of image-sets, each corresponding to a set of slices from a single CT scan. If an image-set has been annotated by another user in the past hour, it shows the name of the user who made the most recent annotation and the time at which it was submitted. The user also has the option of selecting *auto* in which case the system will direct the user to either the last set he/she annotated, or a random unannotated set. A screen capture of this page is depicted in Fig. 2.

Once the user selects an image-set to annotate, it brings them to the page depicted in Fig. 3. Here, he/she is presented with an image in the center of the screen, with thumbnails of the features already annotated below it, and a toolbar above it. Among the tools are *previous* and *next* buttons, a bar of small thumbnails of each slice to choose from, and *submit* buttons for each feature. The user may use the *bucket icon* to switch his/her tool to a bucket fill, or simply by right clicking which also performs this action.

The platform makes use of the CSS3 *filter* element to adjust its brightness and contrast. Medical experts have particular preferences for brightness and contrast for CT images that depend on which part of the body it depicts, and which organs they are studying. We selected abdomen brightness and contrast values (170% and 300%, respectively) by iteratively adjusting and getting feedback from expert urologists.

For this annotation task, we would like segmentation data for five regions of interest: left kidney, right kidney, left mass, right mass, and aorta. If a particular region doesn't exist in an image, the user simply omits that submission, or submits a blank canvas. Once an annotation is submitted, it falls to its respective thumbnail under the large image. Until then, those thumbnails remain gray placeholders.

Select an Image Set <small>auto</small>

P002S00	60 Unannotated	0 Pending	0 Valid	0 Flagged	Nick Heller 5 minutes ago	Annotate / Validate
P003S00	269 Unannotated	0 Pending	0 Valid	0 Flagged	Nick Heller 0 minutes ago	Annotate / Validate
P004S00	105 Unannotated	0 Pending	0 Valid	0 Flagged		Annotate / Validate
P006S00	116 Unannotated	0 Pending	0 Valid	0 Flagged		Annotate / Validate

Fig. 2. The leftmost text of an image-set is that image-set ID, the first denoting patient 2, set 0. Next in from the left is a breakdown of the bins each image in the set resides in. Next is the aforementioned notice of recent activity. Finally we have the annotate and validate buttons.

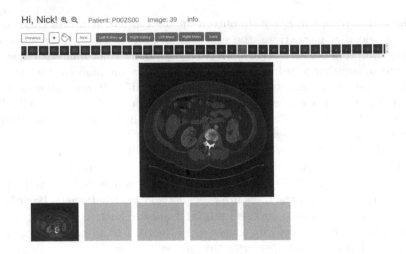

Fig. 3. The interface with which users create their drawn annotations.

The users also have the option to validate annotations. This is a simple binary feedback process on an interface that follows the design of the annotation interface, but instead of five submit buttons, there are only two: accept or reject, after which it stores the response and presents the next annotation. This feature was deployed for ensuring the high quality of the harvested annotations.

4   The Backend

In this section we briefly discuss the backend of this platform. The platform stack is Linux Apache MySQL PHP (LAMP) with some flat files of structured data (JSONs) used for configuration and databasing. The software would likely run slightly faster if the flat files were migrated to MySQL, but as of now, speed is not a major concern.

During annotation, the *brush strokes* and *fill* commands from the user are individually stored locally to allow for undo and redo operations. Once the annotation is submitted, it is stored on the server as a whole image.

5   Evaluation

There are two components to the task of evaluating this platform, namely (i) evaluate the interface of the platform from a general standpoint of interaction design and ease of use, and (ii) evaluate the interface's capacity for allowing users to produce highly accurate image annotations.

5.1   Evaluating Interaction Design and Ease of Use

In addition to the design guidelines given by medical experts during this platform's initial development, we conducted a heuristic evaluation using the Nielsen

Norman Group's 10 heuristics [7]. This technique was selected because it has been shown to be a very effective and low-cost method for identifying weaknesses in a user interface. In that way, the types of flaws that a user study might miss are also identified. As is standard practice, the platform was evaluated by 3 experts trained in heuristic evaluation. Each expert compiled a list of heuristic violations independently. Then, the collected information was consolidated and each violation received and ordinal (0-4) severity score. Those were then averaged to yield the final evaluation score.

Our heuristic evaluation identified 13 violations. Only one violation received a 3, the rest were rated 2 or lower, and highly ranked one was identified as a known issue which at the time of writing was being worked on and near resolution. For brevity, we refrain from listing each violation here, but some clusters we noticed were (i) our platform suffers from the so-called "pottery barn principle" where certain actions have no or limited undo functionality, so users sometimes feel as though they are walking around in a pottery barn, which significantly impairs the user experience, and (ii) our error messages lack informative and constructive feedback about how to proceed in the event of each error. Improvements which address these issues have been slated for development and will likely be deployed a few weeks after writing.

5.2 Evaluating Data Quality

It is important to ensure that the annotations completed with this platform accurately represent the intentions of the expert performing them. We identified region size as a factor which impacts annotation precision. Towards developing size guidelines for freehand annotations, we performed a study in which a single user annotated the same kidney 16 times at each of 8 different levels of zoom. In addition to the annotations, we recorded the time of continuous annotation that the user took during each of the sessions.

To measure precision, for every possible pair in the 16 annotations, we computed the proportion of pixels that are highlighted in one annotation but not in the other, to the number of pixels highlighted in the union of the annotations. We multiplied this by 100 and computed the mean over all pairs which we interpret as the average percentage of deviation at a given level of zoom. The results of this study are shown in Fig. 4.

Our results suggest that there is an inverse correlation between the size of the feature on the screen and the users' error in consistently annotating that feature. The near-highest level of consistency can be seen to occur at feature sizes larger than 10 cm. Further, there appears to be a positive correlation between the size of the feature and the average annotation time.

The focus of this work was to construct a platform for distributing the annotation load across different locations. We wanted to achieve this in such a way that minimized the time elapsed for the pertinent tasks to the annotation. These include saving the annotations properly, and finding and opening the next image. These tasks are cumbersome in the existing more general-purpose GNU Image Manipulation Program (GIMP). In a similar experiment with the same user, we

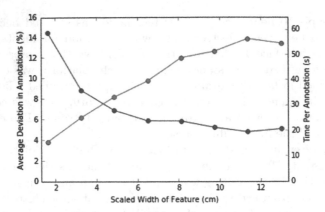

Fig. 4. The downward sloping line (blue) corresponds to the left y-axis and the upward sloping line (red) corresponds to the right y-axis. This chart suggests that for the task of highlighting kidneys, increasing the size of the kidney on the screen up to about 10 cm will improve the annotation consistency, but beyond that, little to no further gains can be made. (Color figure online)

found the mean annotation time using GIMP to be ∼106 s per region of interest at a scaled width of 8.125 cm and ∼123 s per region of interest at a scaled width of 11.375 cm. This suggests that our platform provides a 54% time improvement over GIMP, while no significant difference in consistency was found.

In order to better understand the nature of the deviations, we conducted a follow-up study in which a user who was not familiar with the previous experiment selected a level of zoom at which he/she felt comfortable to perform accurate annotations, and provided 60 annotations of the same feature. A visualization of these annotations are shown in Fig. 5. This user was instructed to focus only on annotation consistency and told that time was not a factor.

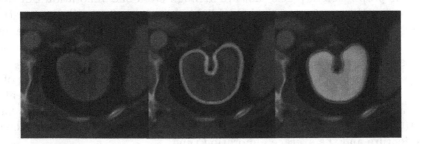

Fig. 5. The background of each image is identical. The left has no overlay, the right is overlaid with each pixel's variance, and the right is overlaid with each pixel's mean. The color-map used is OpenCV's COLORMAP_HOT. We omit a numerical scale since the translucent overlay invalidates any correspondence and the figure is only intended to show a trend. (Color figure online)

The level of zoom that the user selected corresponded to a feature width of less than 4 cm, and that user was very surprised to find that annotations varied, on average, by 11%. This suggests that users' intuition is not accurate at guessing the expected consistency amongst annotations, and that such evaluation studies are deemed necessary prior to investing large amounts of resources in labeling.

6 Future Work

In the near future we intend to release this project as open source software so that other groups can install and serve the platform for their own research purposes. Before we do this, however, there are a number of scheduled improvements to both code clarity and the platform itself.

6.1 UI Improvements

A limited number of potential improvements in the appearance and interaction patterns have been identified from both the heuristic evaluation and the user studies conducted. Most of those could be addressed with relatively little development time. The improvements we intend to make include (i) making the interface more conducive to annotating highly zoomed images, (ii) modifying error messages to be more informative and constructive, (iii) introducing additional functionality to enable users to undo/redo pieces of their brush strokes individually, and (iv) extending the platform such that new annotation projects can be added with a simple addition to a configuration file.

6.2 Added Functionality

The main focus of this work is to reduce the time required by experts to annotate regions of interest. With that in mind, we plan studying the possibility of developing schemes which suggest annotations for each region of interest. These would then be further tuned by the experts, rather than requiring the experts to start drawing from scratch, as implemented in the present version.

Furthermore, the development and evaluation of a system which offers a number of different annotation suggestions and asks the user to select the best among them, is under construction. This process could iterate until the expert is satisfied with the suggestion windows provided by the tool. Heuristically we believe that either of these schemes, or a combination of the two, would result in a significant time improvement over the current method, without compromising the annotation quality.

6.3 Further Evaluation of Annotation Quality

It is imperative that we not only ensure that annotations are performed quickly, but also that they accurately reflect the features they are attempting to segment. We plan to further study this issue through large scale auditing throughout the annotation process. Certain randomly selected image-sets will be duplicated and blindly assigned to additional users to evaluate consistency and identify any biases that certain annotators might hold. This work will further inform our development efforts to mitigate this issue moving forward.

6.4   Utilizing 3D Information

When paired with the annotation data–or conceivably, the segmentations produced by our network–the marching cubes [10] algorithm can be used to create a 3D reconstruction of the features. This reconstruction could be useful for informing treatment decisions or for giving surgeons a better visualization of an area they may be preparing to operate on. We wrote an offline script which, given these annotations, creates this reconstruction. An example is shown in Fig. 6.

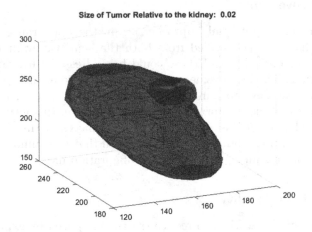

Fig. 6. A 3D reconstruction of a kidney (blue) and tumor (red) based on annotations of slices using our system. (Color figure online)

We plan to further explore ways to present these reconstructions to medical professionals so as to maximize their utility. One idea is to integrate this presentation into the current interface using the WebGL library. Another is to import our meshes into a virtual reality platform.

Acknowledgments. We thank Maxwell Fite and Stamatios Morellas for their expertise on heuristic evaluation, Drs. Christopher Weight, Niranjan Sathianathen, and Suprita Krishna for their feedback on the initial development process, and Samit Roy, Meera Sury, and Michael Tradewell for annotations completed thus far. "'This material is partially based upon work supported by the National Science Foundation through grants #CNS-0934327, #CNS-1039741, #SMA-1028076, #CNS-1338042, #CNS-1439728, #OISE-1551059, and #CNS-1514626.'"

References

1. Russell, B.C., Torralba, A., Murphy, K.P., Freeman, W.T.: LabelMe: a database and web-based tool for image annotation. Int. J. Comput. Vis. **77**, 157–173 (2008)
2. Shehata, M., Khalifa, F., Soliman, A., Abou El-Ghar, M., Dwyer, A., Gimelfarb, G., Keynton, R., El-Baz, A.: A promising non-invasive cad system for kidney function assessment. In: Ourselin, S., Joskowicz, L., Sabuncu, M., Unal, G., Wells, W. (eds.) MICCAI 2016. LNCS, vol. 9902, pp. 613–621. Springer, Cham (2016)
3. Dhungel, N., Carneiro, G., Bradley, A.P.: The automated learning of deep features for breast mass classification from mammograms. In: Ourselin, S., Joskowicz, L., Sabuncu, M.R., Unal, G., Wells, W. (eds.) MICCAI 2016. LNCS, vol. 9901, pp. 106–114. Springer, Cham (2016). doi:10.1007/978-3-319-46723-8_13
4. Wang, J., MacKenzie, J.D., Ramachandran, R., Chen, D.Z.: A deep learning approach for semantic segmentation in histology tissue images. In: Ourselin, S., Joskowicz, L., Sabuncu, M.R., Unal, G., Wells, W. (eds.) MICCAI 2016. LNCS, vol. 9901, pp. 176–184. Springer, Cham (2016). doi:10.1007/978-3-319-46723-8_21
5. Xu, T., Zhang, H., Huang, X., Zhang, S., Metaxas, D.N.: Multimodal deep learning for cervical dysplasia diagnosis. In: Ourselin, S., Joskowicz, L., Sabuncu, M.R., Unal, G., Wells, W. (eds.) MICCAI 2016. LNCS, vol. 9901, pp. 115–123. Springer, Cham (2016). doi:10.1007/978-3-319-46723-8_14
6. Xu, Y., Li, Y., Liu, M., Wang, Y., Lai, M., Chang, E.I.-C.: Gland instance segmentation by deep multichannel side supervision. In: Ourselin, S., Joskowicz, L., Sabuncu, M.R., Unal, G., Wells, W. (eds.) MICCAI 2016. LNCS, vol. 9901, pp. 496–504. Springer, Cham (2016). doi:10.1007/978-3-319-46723-8_57
7. Nielsen, J.: Enhancing the explanatory power of usability heuristics. In: Proceedings of ACM CHI 1994 Conference, pp. 152–158 (1994)
8. CAMELYON16, ISBI challenge on cancer metastasis detection in lymph node. https://camelyon16.grand-challenge.org/
9. Multimodal brain tumor segmentation challenge 2017. http://braintumor segmentation.org/
10. Lorensen, W., Cline, H.: Marching cubes: a high resolution 3D surface reconstruction algorithm. In: Proceedings of SIGGRAPH 1987, vol. 21, pp. 163–169 (1987)

Training Deep Convolutional Neural Networks with Active Learning for Exudate Classification in Eye Fundus Images

Sebastian Otálora[2(✉)], Oscar Perdomo[1], Fabio González[1], and Henning Müller[2]

[1] Universidad Nacional de Colombia, Bogotá, Colombia
[2] University of Applied Sciences Western Switzerland (HES-SO), Sierre, Switzerland
juan.otaloramontenegro@hevs.ch

Abstract. Training deep convolutional neural network for classification in medical tasks is often difficult due to the lack of annotated data samples. Deep convolutional networks (CNN) has been successfully used as an automatic detection tool to support the grading of diabetic retinopathy and macular edema. Nevertheless, the manual annotation of exudates in eye fundus images used to classify the grade of the DR is very time consuming and repetitive for clinical personnel. Active learning algorithms seek to reduce the labeling effort in training machine learning models. This work presents a label-efficient CNN model using the expected gradient length, an active learning algorithm to select the most informative patches and images, converging earlier and to a better local optimum than the usual SGD (Stochastic Gradient Descent) strategy. Our method also generates useful masks for prediction and segments regions of interest.

1 Introduction

Diabetes Mellitus is one of the leading causes of death according to statistics of the World Health Organization.[1] Diabetic Retinopathy (DR) is a condition caused by prolonged diabetes, causing blindness in persons at a relatively young age (20–69 years). The problem is that most persons have no symptoms and suffer the disease without a timely diagnosis. Because the retina is vulnerable to microvascular changes of diabetes and because diabetic retinopathy is the most common complication of diabetes, eye fundus imaging is considered a non-invasive and painless route to screen and monitor DR [6,12].

In the earliest stage of DR, small areas of inflammation called *exudates* appear in the retinal blood vessels, the detection of these yellowish areas that grow along the retina surface is an important step for the ophthalmologist to grade the stage of DR. The manual segmentation of exudates in eye fundus images, is very time consuming and repetitive for clinical personnel [6].

In recent years, deep learning techniques have increased the performance of computer vision systems, deep convolutional neural networks (CNN) were used

---

[1] http://www.who.int/diabetes/en/.

© Springer International Publishing AG 2017
M.J. Cardoso et al. (Eds.): CVII-STENT/LABELS 2017, LNCS 10552, pp. 146–154, 2017.
DOI: 10.1007/978-3-319-67534-3_16

to classify natural images and recognize digits and are now being used successfully in biomedical imaging and computer-aided diagnosis (CADx) systems [3].

CNN models play a major role in DR grading showing superior performance in several settings and datasets compared to previous approaches. In 2015, the data science competition platform Kaggle launched a DR Detection competition[2]. The winner and the top participants used CNNs on more than 35,000 labeled images, demonstrating that for a successful training of such algorithms a significant amount of labeled data is required. In [4] the authors used more than 100,000 labeled eye fundus images to train a CNN with a performance comparable to an ophthalmologist panel. This presents a challenge, as the algorithms need to be fed with in the order of thousand of samples, which in practice is both time-consuming and expensive. It is important to make well-performing algorithms such as CNN less data intensive and thus able to learn with a few selected examples. This is more realistic in clinical practice, also because imaging devices change over time.

Active learning is an important area of machine learning research [10] where the premise is that a machine learning algorithm can achieve good accuracy with fewer training labels if the algorithm chooses the data from which it learns intelligently. This idea is key for building more efficient CADx systems and for reducing costs in building medical image datasets [13] where the expert annotations are costly and time-consuming.

In [14], an active learning algorithm for convolutional deep belief networks is presented with an application to sentiment classification of documents. In [2], the authors show how to formally measure the expected change of model outputs for Gaussian process regression showing an improvement in the area under the ROC curve with fewer queries to the model than the usual random selection. Active learning has also been applied to reduce the number of labeled samples in training CAD systems for DR. Sánchez et al. [9] compare two active leaning approaches, uncertainty sampling and query-by-bagging, showing that with the former, just a reduced number of labeled samples is necessary for the system to achieve a performance of 0.8 in area under the receiving operating characteristic curve. Nevertheless, this approach is computationally intensive for deep CNNs because it is based on building multiple committees of classifiers to choose the most informative sample, which translates into training multiple deep CNNs.

In this work we present a novel approach to detect exudates and highlight the most interesting areas of the eye fundus images using an active learning algorithm called *expected gradient length* (EGL) that works jointly with the CNN model parameters to select the most informative patches and images to train without a significant compromise in the model performance. Our method has the advantage of computing a single backward-forward pass in order to obtain the samples that lead to the most changes in the network parameters, i.e. the most informative images and patches to learn. To the best of our knowledge, this is the first time that an active learning method that uses the deep learning model parameters to select the most relevant samples is presented in the medical imaging field.

---

[2] https://www.kaggle.com/c/diabetic-retinopathy-detection.

2   Deep Learning Model

Convolutional Neural Networks (CNN) are a particular kind of a supervised multi layer perceptrons inspired by the visual cortex. The CNNs are able to detect visual patterns with minimal preprocessing. They are trained with the robustness to respond to the distortion, variability and invariance to the exact position of the pattern and benefit from data augmentation that uses subtle transforms of the input for learning invariances. CNN models are one of the most successful deep learning models for computer vision. The medical imaging field is rapidly adapting these models to solve and improve a plethora of applications [3].

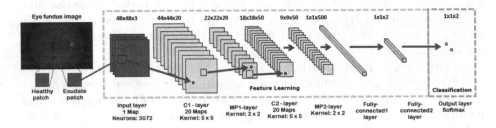

Fig. 1. Deep CNN architecture to classify between healthy and exudate patches.

Our deep learning model is based on a CNN architecture called LeNet [7] with 7 layers as shown in Fig. 1, which is composed of a patch input layer followed by two convolutions and max pooling operations to finalize in a softmax classification layer that outputs the probability of a patch being healthy or exudate. We choose this architecture because of its good classification performance with small input and because (as seen in Sect. 3) our model selects the samples by performing a forward-backward pass over the net. A deeper network would put a computational burden on our experiments.

3   EGL for Patch and Image Selection in Convolutional Neural Networks

Traditional supervised learning algorithms use whatever labeled data is provided to induce a model. Active learning, in contrast, gives the learner a degree of control by allowing to select which instances are labeled and added to the training set. A typical active learner begins with a small labeled set $\mathcal{L}$, selects one or more informative instances from a large unlabeled pool $\mathcal{U}$, learns from these labeled queries (that are added to $\mathcal{L}$), and repeats until convergence. The principle behind active learning is that a machine learning algorithm can achieve similar or even better accuracy when trained with few training labels than with the full training set if the algorithm is allowed to choose the data from which it learns [10].

An active learner may pose queries, usually in the form of unlabeled data instances to be labeled by an oracle (e.g. an ophthalmologist annotator). Active learning is well-motivated in many modern machine learning problems, where unlabeled data may be abundant or easily obtained but labels are not. This is an interesting direction for the so-called *deep learning in the small data regime*, where the objective is to train time-consuming and high sample complexity algorithms with fewer resources, as in the case of medical images.

Stochastic Gradient Descent (SGD) works by stochastically optimizing an objective function J with respect to the model parameters θ. This means to find the model parameters by optimizing with only one sample or sample batches instead of the full training dataset:

$$\theta_{t+1} = \theta_t - \eta \nabla J_i(\theta_t)$$

where $J_i(\theta_t)$ is the objective function evaluated at the i-th sample tuple (x^i, y^i) at iteration t, η is the learning rate and ∇ is the gradient operator. For computing $\nabla J_i(\theta)$ we need the i-th sample representation and its corresponding label, if we measure the norm of this term, i.e. the gradient length term $\|\nabla J_i(\theta)\|$, this quantifies how much the i-th sample and its label contribute to each component of the gradient vector.

A natural choice for selecting the most informative patches for each batch iteration of SGD is to select the instances that give the highest values for the gradient length weighted by the probability of this sample having the y^i label. In other words, to select the instances that create the largest change to the current model if we knew their labels:

$$\Phi(x^i) = \sum_{j=1}^{c} p(y^i = j | x^i) \|\nabla J_i(\theta)\| \tag{1}$$

where c is the total number of labels or classes. The Expected Gradient Length (EGL) works by sorting the Φ values from an unlabeled pool of samples and then adding them to the training dataset by asking an oracle to give the ground truth label of these samples. The EGL algorithm was first mentioned by Settles et al. [11] in the setting of multiple-instance active learning. To the best of our knowledge this is the first time the approach is used in the selection of samples in CNN. For being able to select the most informative samples in a CNN architecture we have to compute the two terms involved in equation (1). For the probability of a sample having the j-th label we can perform a forward propagation through the network and obtain the corresponding probabilities from the softmax layer of the network. To measure the gradient length we can perform a backward propagation through the network to measure the frobenius norm of the gradient parameters. In a CNN architecture we have the flexibility to compute the backward/forward phases up to a certain layer. In our experiments we made the backward down to the first fully connected layer as experiments showed no significant differences for in between layers. This process has to be done over all possible labels for each sample. Once we have computed the Φ

values for all samples, we sort them and select the k samples with the highest EGL values.

Algorithm 1. EGL for Active Selection of patches in a CNN

Require: Patch Dataset $\mathcal{L}$, Initial Trained Model **M** with patches in $\mathcal{L}' \subset \mathcal{L}$, Number k of most informative patches

1: **while** not converged **do**
2:    Create and shuffle batches from $\mathcal{L}$
3:    **for** each batch **do**
4:       Compute $\Phi(x)$ using $\mathbf{M}, \forall x \in$ batch
5:    **end for**
6:    Sort all the Φ values and return the highest k corresponding samples $\mathcal{L}_k$
7:    Update **M** using $\mathcal{L}' \cup \mathcal{L}_k$
8: **end while**

We begin with a small portion of labeled samples $\mathcal{L}' \subset \mathcal{L}$ to train an initial model **M**, and then incrementally adding the k samples to $\mathcal{L}'$ to update **M** parameters. We stop the training procedure when the algorithm converges i.e. when the training and validation errors do not decrease significantly or when the performance in terms of accuracy stays the same for more than one epoch. Since we are able to compute the most significant patches it is straightforward to extend the procedure to select not only the most informative patches but also the most informative images within the training set. The modification is that instead of computing the EGL values for all ground truth exudate and healthy patches we compute the *interestingness* of an image by *patchifying* the image with a given stride and then densely computing Φ. Then, images are sorted by their top EGL values and finally, the patches that belong to the most interesting image are added to the training set for further parameter updates using Algorithm 1 until convergence. We think that this is a more realistic scenario where an ophthalmologist does not have the time to manually annotate all images but only those that contain most information to train a label efficient system. The full algorithm is described in Algorithm 2.

4   Experimental Setup

4.1   Ophtha Dataset

The e-ophtha database with color fundus images was used in this work. The database contains 315 images with a size ranging from 1440×960 to 2540×1690 pixels, 268 images have no lesion and 47 contain exudates that were segmented by ophthalmologists from the OPHDIAT Tele-medical network under a French Research Agency (ANR) project [1]. The labeled patch dataset was created with cropped 48×48 pixel patches that contain both exudate and healthy examples. We prevent over–fitting artificially creating new samples by generating artificially

7 new label-preserving samples using a combination of flipping and 90, 180 and 270° rotations. After the preprocessing steps of cropping and data augmentation, the dataset splits were built with randomly selected patches of each class as follows: a training split with 8760 patches for each class, a validation split with 328 per class and a test split with 986. Images of a given patient could only belong to a single group according to the described dataset distribution. At test time, only patches of unseen patient images are evaluated.

4.2 Evaluation

The technique of Decencieriere et al. [1] was chosen as our baseline. The base LeNet model was trained using stochastic gradient descent (SGD) from scratch without any transfer learning from other datasets. The learning rate and batch size were explored in a grid search and showed robustness in the range of 32–64 in terms of batch size with a learning rate of 0.01 when trained with all the training patches. In our final experiments we set the batch size to 32 and 0.01 for the learning rate, using 30 as the number of epochs to train the model. The model M is the LeNet CNN model described in Fig. 1 and initially trained with 5 batches of 32 samples.

The proposed approach was implemented in Python 2.7 and the Caffe deep learning framework [5] that allows for efficient access to parameters and data in memory. We use an NVIDIA GTX TITANX GPU for our experiments. During all the experiments, training loss, validation loss, as well as the accuracy over the validation set were monitored.

5 Results

We test our Algorithm 2 in the scenario where an ophthalmologist selects only a few important or relevant images instead of patches to annotate and train

---

Algorithm 2. EGL for Active Selection of images in a Convolutional Neural Network.

Require: Training Image Set $\mathcal{T}$, Patch Dataset $\mathcal{L}$, Number μ of initial images to look at

    Select an initial set $\mathcal{T}_\mu$ of images randomly

2: Train initial model M using the ground truth patches from the μ images

    while not converged **do**

4:     **for** each image in $\mathcal{T} \setminus \mathcal{T}_\mu$ **do**

        Patchify image and compute $\sigma_{image} = \displaystyle\sum_{patch \in image} \Phi(patch)$, using M

6:     **end for**

    Sort all the σ_{image} values and return $\mathcal{I}_{max}$, the image with higher sum

8:     $\mathcal{T}_\mu = \mathcal{T}_\mu \cup \mathcal{I}_{max}$

    $\mathcal{L}_\mu = \{ \text{patch} \in \mathcal{L}_\mathcal{I}, \forall \mathcal{I} \in \mathcal{T}_\mu \}$

10:     Update M with k selected patches using Algorithm 1 and the patches in $\mathcal{L}_\mu$

    end while

---

the model. In Fig. 2 the left side of the orange line is when the initial model training is performed. Then, the Algorithm 2 is used to select the most interesting image for the model and subsequently to update the model. In our approach, the convergence is reached at an earlier stage. As few as 15 batches are enough for the model convergence, showing that in this more realistic scenario our strategy also outperforms the standard way of training deep CNN models.

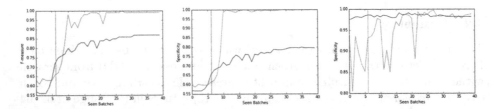

Fig. 2. Results for F-Measure, sensitivity and specificity, using the random strategy (blue) and active learning using EGL (green) for Algorithm 2. In this setup only the patches of the 4 initial training images were used for training the model in the first 6 SGD iterations, after this (orange line) we add the patches from the images with maximum EGL value to the training set. (Color figure online)

Once we have an initial training of the model we can measure the interestingness of a full image computing the sum of its EGL values. This was the criterion to select images for the results of Algorithm 2. An example image with its interestingness values over different training times is shown in Fig. 2. We can plot this value and see how this evolves as the model sees more batches. These values are illustrated in Fig. 3. Here we can see how the interestingness value decays after the model has converged, so when the loss function does not decrease anymore and the norm of the parameters is nearly 0.

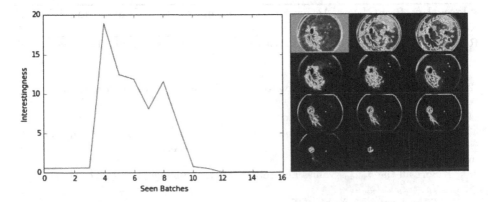

Fig. 3. Interestingness over training time. After the model converges the interestingness value decays to 0 because the norm of the gradient is close to 0.

6   Discussion

This paper presents for the first time an active learning strategy to select the most relevant samples and images for a sample efficient training of a deep convolutional neural network to classify exudate patterns in eye fundus images. The proposed strategy was able to achieve a similar performance compared to the model trained with the full dataset [8] but only using an informative portion of the training data. Besides the speed-up for convergence, our algorithm also brings an additional interpretation layer for deep CNN models that locates the regions of the image that the ophthalmologist should label, improving the interaction between the model and the specialist that conventional CNN models lack. Our approach presents a computational drawback when the number of unlabeled data–samples to check is large, but we think that this could be overcome with traditional sampling techniques. Despite our results showing good performance using only a portion of the data, we would like to do further experimentation using only the initially labeled portion and involving large–scale datasets where the combination of our sample selection techniques with transfer learning could lead to a performance boost. We think that active learning techniques have a promising application landscape in the challenging tasks of medical imaging using deep learning because of their potential to relief the need for large amounts of labeled data. This will allow the usage of deep learning models in a broader set of medical imaging tasks like detection and segmentation of structures in specialized domains such as histopathology image analysis or computed tomography scans where the labels are costly.

Acknowledgments. This work was supported by the Administrative Department of Science, Technology and Innovation of Colombia (Colciencias) through the grant Jóvenes Investigadores 2014 in call 645 and by Nvidia with a TitanX GPU.

References

1. Decencière, E., Cazuguel, G., Zhang, X., Thibault, G., Klein, J.C., Meyer, F., Marcotegui, B., Quellec, G., Lamard, M., Danno, R., et al.: Teleophta: machine learning and image processing methods for teleophthalmology. IRBM **34**(2), 196–203 (2013)
2. Freytag, A., Rodner, E., Denzler, J.: Selecting influential examples: active learning with expected model output changes. In: Fleet, D., Pajdla, T., Schiele, B., Tuytelaars, T. (eds.) ECCV 2014. LNCS, vol. 8692, pp. 562–577. Springer, Cham (2014). doi:10.1007/978-3-319-10593-2_37
3. Greenspan, H., van Ginneken, B., Summers, R.M.: Guest editorial deep learning in medical imaging: overview and future promise of an exciting new technique. IEEE Trans. Med. Imaging **35**(5), 1153–1159 (2016)
4. Gulshan, V., Peng, L., Coram, M., Stumpe, M.C., Wu, D., Narayanaswamy, A., Venugopalan, S., Widner, K., Madams, T., Cuadros, J., et al.: Development and validation of a deep learning algorithm for detection of diabetic retinopathy in retinal fundus photographs. JAMA **316**(22), 2402–2410 (2016)

5. Jia, Y., Shelhamer, E., Donahue, J., Karayev, S., Long, J., Girshick, R., Guadarrama, S., Darrell, T.: Caffe: convolutional architecture for fast feature embedding. In: Proceedings of the 22nd ACM International Conference on Multimedia, pp. 675–678. ACM (2014)
6. Kauppi, T., et al.: Eye fundus image analysis for automatic detection of diabetic retinopathy. Lappeenranta University of Technology (2010)
7. LeCun, Y., Bottou, L., Bengio, Y., Haffner, P.: Gradient-based learning applied to document recognition. Proc. IEEE 86(11), 2278–2324 (1998)
8. Perdomo, O., Otalora, S., Rodríguez, F., Arevalo, J., González, F.A.: A novel machine learning model based on exudate localization to detect diabetic macular edema. In: Ophthalmic Medical Image Analysis Third International Workshop (OMIA 2016), pp. 137–144. University of Iowa (2016)
9. Sánchez, C.I., Niemeijer, M., Abràmoff, M.D., van Ginneken, B.: Active learning for an efficient training strategy of computer-aided diagnosis systems: application to diabetic retinopathy screening. In: Jiang, T., Navab, N., Pluim, J.P.W., Viergever, M.A. (eds.) MICCAI 2010. LNCS, vol. 6363, pp. 603–610. Springer, Heidelberg (2010). doi:10.1007/978-3-642-15711-0_75
10. Settles, B.: Active learning literature survey. Univ. Wis. Madison 52(55–66), 11 (2010)
11. Settles, B., Craven, M., Ray, S.: Multiple-instance active learning. In: Advances in Neural Information Processing Systems, pp. 1289–1296 (2008)
12. Stitt, A.W., Lois, N., Medina, R.J., Adamson, P., Curtis, T.M.: Advances in our understanding of diabetic retinopathy. Clin. Sci. 125(1), 1–17 (2013)
13. Yu, F., Seff, A., Zhang, Y., Song, S., Funkhouser, T., Xiao, J.: LSUN: construction of a large-scale image dataset using deep learning with humans in the loop. arXiv preprint arXiv:1506.03365 (2015)
14. Zhou, S., Chen, Q., Wang, X.: Active semi-supervised learning method with hybrid deep belief networks. PLoS ONE 9(9), e107122 (2014)

Uncertainty Driven Multi-loss Fully Convolutional Networks for Histopathology

Aïcha BenTaieb$^{(\boxtimes)}$ and Ghassan Hamarneh

Medical Image Analysis Lab, School of Computing Science,
Simon Fraser University, Burnaby, Canada
{abentaie,hamarneh}@sfu.ca

Abstract. Different works have shown that the combination of multiple loss functions is beneficial when training deep neural networks for a variety of prediction tasks. Generally, such multi-loss approaches are implemented via a weighted multi-loss objective function in which each term encodes a different desired inference criterion. The importance of each term is often set using empirically tuned hyper-parameters. In this work, we analyze the importance of the relative weighting between the different terms of a multi-loss function and propose to leverage the model's uncertainty with respect to each loss as an automatically learned weighting parameter. We consider the application of colon gland analysis from histopathology images for which various multi-loss functions have been proposed. We show improvements in classification and segmentation accuracy when using the proposed uncertainty driven multi-loss function.

1 Introduction

Although deep learning models have shown remarkable results on a variety of prediction tasks, recent works applied to medical image analysis have demonstrated improved performance by incorporating additional domain-specific information [1]. In fact, medical image analysis datasets are typically not large enough for learning robust features, however, there exist a variety of expert knowledge that can be leveraged to guide the underlying learning model. Such knowledge or cues are generally considered as a set of auxiliary losses that serve to improve or guide the learning of a primary task (e.g. image classification or segmentation). Specifically, these cues are incorporated in the training of deep convolutional networks using a multi-loss objective function combining a variety of objectives learned from a shared image representation. The combination of multiple loss functions can be interpreted as a form of regularization as it constrains search space for possible candidate solutions for the primary task.

Different types of cues can be combined in a multi-loss objective function to improve the generalization of deep networks. Multi-loss functions have been proposed for a variety of medical applications: colon histology images, skin dermoscopy images or chest X-Ray images. Chen et al. [2] proposed a multi-loss learning framework for gland segmentation from histology images in which features from different layers of a deep fully convolutional network were combined

© Springer International Publishing AG 2017
M.J. Cardoso et al. (Eds.): CVII-STENT/LABELS 2017, LNCS 10552, pp. 155–163, 2017.
DOI: 10.1007/978-3-319-67534-3_17

through auxiliary loss functions and added to a per-pixel classification loss. Ben-Taieb et al. [3] proposed a two-loss objective function combining gland classification (malignant vs benign) and segmentation (gland delineation) and showed that both tasks were mutually beneficial. Additionally, authors also proposed a multi-loss objective function for gland segmentation that equips a fully convolutional network with topological and geometrical constraints [4] that encourage learning topologically plausible and smooth segmentations. Kawahara et al. [5] used auxiliary losses to train a multi-scale convolutional network to classify skin lesions. More recently, adversarial loss functions were also proposed as additional forms of supervision. Dai et al. [6] leveraged an adversarial loss to guide the segmentation of organs from chest X-Ray images. While these previous works confirm the utility of training deep networks with a multi-loss objective function, they do not clearly explain how to set the contribution of each loss.

Most existing works use an empirical approach to combine different losses. Generally, all losses are simply summed with equal contribution or manually tuned hyper-parameters are used to control the trade-off among all terms. In this work, we investigate the importance of an appropriate choice of weighting between each loss and propose a way to automate it. Specifically, we utilize concepts from Bayesian deep learning [7,8] and introduce an uncertainty based multi-loss objective function. In the proposed multi-loss, the importance of each term is learned based on the model's uncertainty with respect to each loss. Uncertainty was leveraged in many medical image analysis applications (e.g. segmentation [9], registration [10]). However, to the best of our knowledge, uncertainty was only explored for the task of image registration in the context of deep learning models for medical images. Yang et al. [11] proposed a CNN model for image registration and showed how uncertainty helps highlighting misaligned regions. Previous works did not consider automating or using uncertainty for guiding the training of multi-loss objective functions designed for medical image analysis.

We illustrate our approach on the task of colon gland analysis leveraging the multi-loss objective functions proposed in previous works [3,4]. We extend these previous works by re-defining the proposed loss functions with an uncertainty driven weighting. We linearly combine classification, segmentation, topology and geometry losses weighted by the model's uncertainty for each of these terms. In the proposed uncertainty driven multi-loss, the uncertainty captures how much variance there is in the model's predictions. This variance or noise in the predictions varies for each term and thus reflects the uncertainty inherent to the classification, segmentation, topology or geometry loss.

Our contributions in this work can be summarized as follows: (i) we show how uncertainty can be used to guide the optimization of multi-loss deep networks in an end-to-end trainable framework; (ii) we combine a series of objectives that have been shown successful for gland analysis and adapt them to encode uncertainty driven weighting; (iii) we analyze the influence of different trade-offs controlling the importance of each loss in a multi-loss objective function and draw some conclusions on the adaptability of neural networks.

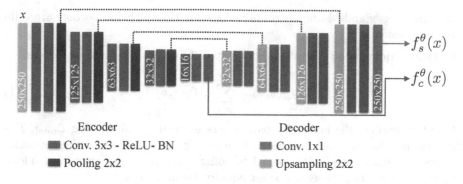

Fig. 1. Multi-loss network architecture. We use an encoder-decoder architecture with skip connections [12]. x is an input image. $f_c^\theta(x)$ are the activations from the last convolution layer of the encoder and are used to predict class labels (i.e. malignant vs benign tissue). $f_s^\theta(x)$ are per-pixel activations from the last convolutional layer of the decoder that are used to predict segmentations. The building blocks of the network are layers of convolution (Conv.), ReLU activation functions and batch normalization (BN). Dashed lines represent skip connections.

2   Method

Our goal is to learn how to combine multiple terms relevant to gland image analysis into a single objective function. For instance, gland classification and gland segmentation can both benefit from a joint learning framework and information about the geometry and topology of glands can facilitate learning plausible segmentations. Note that we refer to gland's geometry and topology in terms of smooth boundaries as well as containment and exclusion properties between different parts of objects (the lumen is generally contained within a thick epithelial border and surrounded by stroma cells that exclude both the lumen and the border, see Fig. 3 for an example of gland segmentation).

We train a fully convolutional network parameterized by θ, from a set of training images x and their corresponding ground truth segmentation masks S along with their tissue class label binary vector C represented by $\{(x^{(n)}, S^{(n)}, C^{(n)}); n = 1, 2, \ldots, N\}$. We drop (n) when referring to a single image x, class label C or segmentation mask S. We note K the total number of image class labels (e.g. $K = 2$ for malignant or benign tissue images of colon adenocarcinomas) and L the total number of region labels in the segmentation mask (e.g. $L = 3$ for lumen, epithelial border and stroma). The network's architecture is shown in Fig. 1. To predict class labels C, we use the network's activations $f_c^\theta(x)$ from the last layer of the encoder as they correspond to a coarser representation of x. To obtain a crisp segmentation of a color image x, we use the activations $f_s^\theta(x)$ from the last layer of the decoder and we assign a vector $S_p = (S_p^1, S_p^2, \ldots, S_p^L) \in \{0, 1\}^L$ to the p-th pixel x_p in x, where S_p^r indicates whether pixel x_p belongs to region r, and L is the number of region labels. We assume region labels r are not always mutually exclusive such that containment properties (e.g. glands' lumen is contained within the epithelial border) are valid label assignments.

Multi-loss networks: A multi-loss objective function is defined as follows:

$$\mathcal{L}_{total}(x;\theta) = \sum_{i=1}^{T} \lambda_i \mathcal{L}_i(x;\theta) \tag{1}$$

where θ represents the network's parameters learned by minimizing $\mathcal{L}_{total}$; T is the total number of loss functions $\mathcal{L}_i$ to minimize with respect to the network's parameters, and λ_i is a scalar coefficient controlling the importance of each loss, generally found via grid-search or set equally for all terms.

In the context of gland analysis, we define a multi-loss objective function that encodes classification, segmentation as well as gland's topology and geometry. We learn the relative weights of each term in the objective using a measure of uncertainty that reflects the amount of noise or variance in the model's predictions for each term. Using uncertainty to weight each term results in reducing the influence of uncertain terms on the total loss and hence on the model's parameters update. Formally, we write the total objective function as follows:

$$\mathcal{L}_{total}(x;\theta,\sigma_c,\sigma_s,\sigma_t,\sigma_g) = \mathcal{L}_c(x;\theta,\sigma_c) + \mathcal{L}_s(x;\theta,\sigma_s) + \mathcal{L}_t(x;\theta,\sigma_t) + \mathcal{L}_g(x;\theta,\sigma_g) \tag{2}$$

where $\mathcal{L}_c, \mathcal{L}_s, \mathcal{L}_t, \mathcal{L}_g$ are the classification, segmentation, topology and geometry loss functions and $\sigma_c, \sigma_s, \sigma_t, \sigma_g$ are learned scalar values representing the uncertainty for each loss (or amount of variance in the prediction).

Uncertainty guided classification: Similarly to Gal et al. [8], we define the classification loss $\mathcal{L}_c$ with uncertainty as:

$$\mathcal{L}_c(x;\theta,\sigma_c) = \sum_{k=1}^{K} -C_k \log P(C_k = 1|x,\theta,\sigma_c), \quad P(C_k = 1|x,\theta,\sigma_c) = \frac{\exp(\frac{1}{\sigma_c^2} f_{c_k}^{\theta}(x))}{\sum_{k'=1}^{K} \exp(\frac{1}{\sigma_c^2} f_{c_{k'}}^{\theta}(x))} \tag{3}$$

where K is the total number of classes, $P(C_k|x,\theta,\sigma_c)$ corresponds to the softmax function over the network's activations $f_c^{\theta}(x)$ weighted by the classification prediction's uncertainty coefficient σ_c. Note how higher values of σ_c reduce the magnitude of activations $f_c^{\theta}(x)$ over all classes (which corresponds to encouraging uniform probabilities $P(C_k|x,\theta,\sigma_c)$) and thus reflect more uncertain predictions (i.e. high activation values will be weighted lower when σ_c; the uncertainty, is high).

Assuming $\frac{1}{\sigma_c^2} \sum_k \exp\left(\frac{1}{\sigma_c^2} f_{c_k}^{\theta}(x)\right) \approx \left(\sum_k \exp(f_{c_k}^{\theta}(x))\right)^{\frac{1}{\sigma_c^2}}$ [7], we can re-write the uncertainty-guided classification loss as follows:

$$\mathcal{L}_c(x;\theta,\sigma_c) = \sum_{k=1}^{K} -C_k \log\left(\exp(\frac{1}{\sigma_c^2} f_{c_k}^{\theta}(x))\right) + \log \sum_{k'=1}^{K} \exp(\frac{1}{\sigma_c^2} f_{c_{k'}}^{\theta}(x)) \tag{4}$$

$$\approx \frac{1}{\sigma_c^2} \sum_{k=1}^{K} -C_k \log P(C_k = 1|x_p;\theta) + \log \sigma_c^2. \tag{5}$$

Note how large scale values of σ_c^2 corresponding to high uncertainty will reduce the contribution of the classification loss. The second term in Eq. (5) avoids σ_c^2 from becoming infinity and thus avoids the loss from becoming zero. We extend the above softmax with uncertainty cross-entropy classification loss to the segmentation losses.

Uncertainty guided segmentation: We learn pixel-wise predictions using a combination of a sigmoid cross entropy loss $\mathcal{L}_s$ with two higher order penalty terms (proposed in [4]): a topology loss $\mathcal{L}_t$ enforcing a hierarchy between labels and a pairwise loss $\mathcal{L}_g$ enforcing smooth segmentations.

$$\mathcal{L}_s(x;\theta,\sigma_s) = \frac{1}{\sigma_s^2} \sum_{p\in\Omega} \sum_{r=1}^{L} -S_p^r \log P(S_p^r = 1|x,\theta) + \log \sigma_s^2 \tag{6}$$

where L represents the number of regions in the segmentation mask, Ω is the set of pixels in a given image x, $P(S_p^r = 1|x,\theta,\sigma_s)$ is the output of the sigmoid function applied to the segmentation activations $f_s^\theta(x_p)$ and σ_s^2 represents the model's uncertainty for $\mathcal{L}_s$.

The topology loss defined in [4] was originally formulated as a modified softmax cross entropy loss in which the probabilities are defined to encode containment and exclusion as a hierarchy between labels. Per-pixel hierarchical probabilities are defined to penalize topologically incorrect label assignments such that their probability is set to zero. Formally, the hierarchical probabilities used to compute $\mathcal{L}_t$ are defined as:

$$P_t(S_p^r|x_p;\theta) = \frac{1}{Z} V(S_p) \prod_{r=1}^{L} \exp\left(f_{s_r}^\theta(x_p)\right) \times S_p^r, \quad Z = \sum_{r=1}^{L} \tilde{P}_t(S_p^r|x_p;\theta) \tag{7}$$

where Z is a normalizing factor, $\tilde{P}_t(S_p^r|x_p;\theta)$ is the un-normalized probability and $V(S_p)$ is a binary indicator function that identifies topologically valid label assignments ($V(S_p) = 1$) from invalid ones ($V(S_p) = 0$). Using these probabilities defined in [4] and applying the same simplification as in Eq. (5), $\mathcal{L}_t$ is formulated as the following uncertainty guided cross entropy loss where σ_t^2 is the uncertainty:

$$\mathcal{L}_t(x;\theta,\sigma_t) = \frac{1}{\sigma_t^2} \sum_{p\in\Omega} \sum_{r=1}^{L} -S_p^r \log P_t(S_p^r = 1|x,\theta) + \log \sigma_t^2. \tag{8}$$

It is worth noting that the fundamental assumption behind the sigmoid cross entropy loss $\mathcal{L}_s$ is that all segmentation labels are mutually independent whereas in the defined topology loss $\mathcal{L}_t$ inclusion and exclusion relations between the segmentation labels are set as hard constraints (i.e. enforcing containment and exclusion properties). Thus, the combination of $\mathcal{L}_s$ and $\mathcal{L}_t$ results in a soft constraint over the topology properties (as opposed to the hard constraint originally proposed in [4]).

Finally, to include uncertainty in the geometry loss, we re-define the original loss proposed in [4] such that it is weighted with an uncertainty coefficient σ_g.

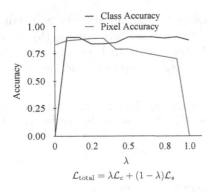
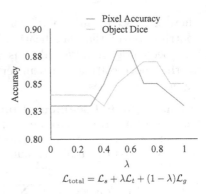

$$\mathcal{L}_{\text{total}} = \lambda \mathcal{L}_c + (1-\lambda)\mathcal{L}_s \qquad\qquad \mathcal{L}_{\text{total}} = \mathcal{L}_s + \lambda \mathcal{L}_t + (1-\lambda)\mathcal{L}_g$$

Fig. 2. Trade-off between different loss functions and influence on the network's generalization. The learning rate was kept fixed to 1e−2 in all experiments. Each graph represents the classification and segmentation accuracy on the Warwick-QU colon adenocarcinoma test set.

The geometry loss $\mathcal{L}_g$ favours smooth segmentations by minimizing the ratio of log probabilities between neighbouring pixels sharing the same labels in the ground truth segmentation.

$$\mathcal{L}_g(x; \theta, \sigma_g) = \frac{1}{\sigma_g^2} \sum_{p \in \Omega} \sum_{r=1}^{L} \sum_{q \in \mathcal{N}^p} S_p^r \left| \log \frac{P_t(S_p^r | x_p; \theta)}{P_t(S_q^r | x_q; \theta)} \right| B_{p,q} + \log \sigma_g^2 \qquad (9)$$

where $\mathcal{N}^p$ corresponds to the 4-connected neighborhood of pixel p. $\mathcal{L}_g$ trains the network to output regularized pairs of log-sigmoid label probabilities for neighbouring pixels p and q when the binary indicator variable $B_{p,q} = 1$ (i.e. when p and q share the same label in the ground truth segmentation). σ_g^2 is the uncertainty for loss $\mathcal{L}_g$. Note that in this formulation, we minimize the difference between log-probabilities so the assumption utilized in Eq. (5) still holds.

Implementation details: We implement the model using Tensorflow [13]. We train a fully convolutional architecture as describe in Fig. 1 using the proposed multi-loss function Eq. (2) optimized with stochastic gradient descent. All uncertainty parameters σ_i are learned along with the model's parameters θ. In practice, we trained the network to predict $\log \sigma_i^2$ for numerical stability [8].

3 Experiments and Discussion

We used the publicly available Warwick-QU colon adenocarcinoma dataset [14], which consists of 85 training (37 benign and 48 malignant) and 80 test images (37 benign and 43 malignant). In this dataset, each tissue image is composed of multiple glands and is labelled as benign or malignant and provided with a corresponding segmentation mask delineating each gland's lumen and epithelial border (see Fig. 3). In all experiments, we used 70 images for training, 15 for validation and 80 for test. We extracted patches of size 250×250 pixels and used a series of elastic and affine transforms to augment the training dataset by a factor of ~100. We used (image-level) classification accuracy to evaluate the model's capacity to correctly predict benign vs malignant tissue images. To evaluate the predicted segmentation masks, we used three different metrics: pixel accuracy to evaluate the accuracy in predicting a pixel as either background, lumen or epithelial border; object Dice and Hausdorff Distance to evaluate the capacity of the model in correctly identifying individual glands in an image. Object Dice and Hausdorff distance are particularly useful in evaluating the accuracy of the predicted segmentations at objects borders.

Table 1. Performance of different loss functions combined with manually tuned loss weights and uncertainty-guided weights. Results are reported on the Warwick-QU original test set.

Loss	Weights				Classification accuracy	Pixel accuracy	Object dice	Hausdorff distance
	$\mathcal{L}_c$	$\mathcal{L}_s$	$\mathcal{L}_t$	$\mathcal{L}_g$				
$\mathcal{L}_c$	1	0	0	0	0.87	–	–	–
$\mathcal{L}_s$	0	1	0	0	–	0.79	0.81	8.2
$\mathcal{L}_t$	0	0	1	0	–	0.75	0.77	8.6
$\mathcal{L}_s + \mathcal{L}_t + \mathcal{L}_g$	0	1	1	1	–	0.83	0.84	7.3
$\mathcal{L}_c + \mathcal{L}_s$	0.5	0.5	0	0	0.90	0.79	0.80	8.4
$\mathcal{L}_c + \mathcal{L}_s + \mathcal{L}_t$	0.33	0.33	0.33	0	0.94	0.78	0.80	8.4
$\mathcal{L}_c + \mathcal{L}_s + \mathcal{L}_t + \mathcal{L}_g$	0.25	0.25	0.25	0.25	0.91	0.81	0.83	7.6
$\mathcal{L}_c + \mathcal{L}_s + \mathcal{L}_t + \mathcal{L}_g$	0.1	0.6	0.22	0.08	**0.95**	**0.86**	0.85	7.1
$\mathcal{L}_c + \mathcal{L}_s$	Trained with uncertainty				**0.95**	0.78	0.80	8.4
$\mathcal{L}_c + \mathcal{L}_s + \mathcal{L}_t$					0.94	0.79	0.81	8.2
$\mathcal{L}_c + \mathcal{L}_s + \mathcal{L}_t + \mathcal{L}_g$					**0.95**	0.85	**0.87**	**7.0**

Multi-loss vs single-loss: We first tested if the combination of different loss functions without uncertainty guidance influences the classification and segmentation accuracy. We used $\mathcal{L}_{\text{total}} = \lambda\mathcal{L}_c + (1 - \lambda)\mathcal{L}_s$ and explored different values for $\lambda \in [0, 1]$. Figure 2 shows the classification as well as the per-pixel accuracy on the Warwick-QU original test set of 80 images for different values of λ. Overall, we observed that learning with multiple losses improved both segmentation and classification performance. In fact, we observed up to 3% (i.e. $\lambda = \{0.5, 0.6, 0.7\}$) increase in classification accuracy when using a combination of $\mathcal{L}_c$ and $\mathcal{L}_s$ compared to using $\mathcal{L}_c$ only (i.e. $\lambda = 1$). Similarly, for segmentation, we observed the performance improved up to 6% (i.e. $\lambda = 0.3$) in pixel accuracy when combining both losses compared to using $\mathcal{L}_s$ only (i.e. $\lambda = 0$). A similar result is shown in Table 1 when comparing $\mathcal{L}_c$ vs $\mathcal{L}_c + \mathcal{L}_s$ with equal weights.

Penalty terms trade-off: We also tested the trade-off between the topology and geometry soft constraints when combined with the segmentation loss. We used different weighting coefficients λ and trained the network with $\mathcal{L}_{\text{total}} = \mathcal{L}_s + \lambda \mathcal{L}_t + (1 - \lambda)\mathcal{L}_g$. We only varied the importance of the soft constraints. It is interesting to note that there is a wide range of weighting coefficients for which the network produces similar (or almost identical) results. In fact, we observed a minimal change ($\leq 1e\text{-}2$) when varying the importance of each term by $\pm 20\%$ around $\lambda = 0.5$, which reflects the flexibility of deep networks to adapt to different regularization terms. We also observed that generally sigmoid cross entropy loss $\mathcal{L}_s$ was more stable than $\mathcal{L}_t$ or $\mathcal{L}_g$-only and outperformed these other losses when each of them was used alone (see Table 1, $\mathcal{L}_s$ only vs $\mathcal{L}_t$ only). However, for certain weighting configurations for each penalty term, we observed improved performance (up to 5%, see Fig. 2) in terms of pixel accuracy and object Dice (e.g. $\lambda = 0.1$ vs. $\lambda = 0.5$).

Uncertainty driven trade-off: To evaluate the utility of using uncertainty to guide the trade-off between the different loss functions, we tested different combinations of losses with uncertainty to form the total multi-loss function. Table 1 shows the performance of each tested loss configuration in terms of class accuracy, pixel accuracy, object Dice and Hausdorff distance. Overall, adding uncertainty to weigh each loss achieves competing results with other strategies (e.g. equally weighted losses) and can even outperform the best set of weights we could find using a finer grid search (in terms of classification accuracy, object Dice and Hausdorff Distance, see Table 1). Note that finding the best set of weights shown in Table 1 involved training more than 30 networks with different weights for each loss whereas using the proposed uncertainty driven weights only involved training a single network. Examples of the segmentation predictions obtained using the proposed method (Eq. 2) are shown in Fig. 3.

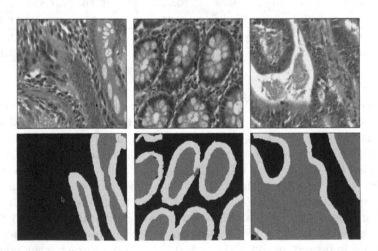

Fig. 3. Examples of predicted segmentations. Colors on the segmentation masks represent gland's central area or lumen (purple), the epithelial border surrounding the lumen (yellow) and the stroma or background (black). (Color figure online)

4   Conclusion

We showed that the combination of different loss terms with appropriate weighting can improve model generalization in the context of deep neural networks. We proposed to use uncertainty as a way to combine multiple loss functions that were shown useful for the analysis of glands in colon adenocarcinoma and we observed that this strategy helps improve classification and segmentation performance and can thus bypass the need for extensive grid-search over different weighting configurations. An interesting extension to our work could be to introduce per-instance uncertainty (as opposed to per-loss) which may be useful in situations where the data or labels are noisy.

References

1. Litjens , G., et al.: A survey on deep learning in medical image analysis. arXiv preprint arXiv:1702.05747 (2017)
2. Chen, H., Qi, X., Yu, L., Heng, P.-A.: DCAN: deep contour-aware networks for accurate gland segmentation. In: Proceedings of the IEEE Conference on Computer Vision and Pattern Recognition, pp. 2487–2496 (2016)
3. BenTaieb, A., Kawahara, J., Hamarneh, G.: Multi-loss convolutional networks for gland analysis in microscopy. In: IEEE 13th International Symposium on Biomedical Imaging, pp. 642–645 (2016)
4. BenTaieb, A., Hamarneh, G.: Topology aware fully convolutional networks for histology gland segmentation. In: Ourselin, S., Joskowicz, L., Sabuncu, M.R., Unal, G., Wells, W. (eds.) MICCAI 2016. LNCS, vol. 9901, pp. 460–468. Springer, Cham (2016). doi:10.1007/978-3-319-46723-8_53
5. Kawahara, J., Hamarneh, G.: Multi-resolution-tract CNN with hybrid pretrained and skin-lesion trained layers. In: Wang, L., Adeli, E., Wang, Q., Shi, Y., Suk, H.-I. (eds.) MLMI 2016. LNCS, vol. 10019, pp. 164–171. Springer, Cham (2016). doi:10.1007/978-3-319-47157-0_20
6. Dai, W., et al.: Scan: structure correcting adversarial network for chest x-rays organ segmentation. arXiv preprint arXiv:1703.08770 (2017)
7. Kendall, A., Gal, Y., Cipolla, R.: Multi-task learning using uncertainty to weigh losses for scene geometry and semantics. arXiv preprint arXiv:1705.07115 (2017)
8. Gal, Y.: Uncertainty in deep learning, Ph.D. dissertation (2016)
9. Saad, A., Möller, T., Hamarneh, G.: Probexplorer: uncertainty-guided exploration and editing of probabilistic medical image segmentation. Comput. Graph. Forum 29(3), 1113–1122 (2010). Wiley Online Library
10. Marsland, S., Shardlow, T.: Langevin equations for landmark image registration with uncertainty. SIAM J. Imaging Sci. 10(2), 782–807 (2017)
11. Yang, X., Kwitt, R., Niethammer, M.: Fast predictive image registration. In: Carneiro, G., et al. (eds.) LABELS/DLMIA -2016. LNCS, vol. 10008, pp. 48–57. Springer, Cham (2016). doi:10.1007/978-3-319-46976-8_6
12. Badrinarayanan, V., Kendall, A., Cipolla, R.: Segnet: a deep convolutional encoder-decoder architecture for scene segmentation. IEEE Trans. Pattern Anal. Mach. Intell. (2017)
13. Abadi, M., et al.: Tensorflow: large-scale machine learning on heterogeneous distributed systems. arXiv preprint arXiv:1603.04467 (2016)
14. Sirinukunwattana, K., et al.: Gland segmentation in colon histology images: the GlaS challenge contest. Med. Image Anal. 35, 489–502 (2017)

Author Index

Printed in the United States
By Bookmasters

Printed in the United States
By Bookmasters